MW01703353

How to Resolve Patient Complaints to Manage Risk

100 of Your Peers' Best Responses

Cindy Ebner, MSN, RN
Angela Burnette, JD
Cristine Vogel, MPH
Nancy Davis, MS, RHIA

HCPro

How to Resolve Patient Complaints to Manage Risk: 100 of your Peers' Best Responses is published by HCPro, Inc.

Copyright 2003 HCPro, Inc.

All rights reserved. Printed in the United States of America. 5 4 3

ISBN 1-57830-357-4

No part of this publication may be reproduced, in any form or by any means, without prior written consent of HCPro or the Copyright Clearance Center (978/750-8400). Please notify us immediately if you have received an unauthorized copy.

HCPro provides information resources for the healthcare industry.

HCPro is not affiliated in any way with the Joint Commission on Accreditation of Healthcare Organizations, which owns the JCAHO trademark.

Julie Pippert, Contributing Writer and Editor
Bryan Cote, Contributing Writer and Editor
Angela Burnette, JD, Contributing Author
Nancy Davis, MS, RHIA, Contributing Author
Cindy Ebner, MSN, RN, Contributing Author
Cristine Vogel, MPH, Contributing Author
Jean St. Pierre, Director of Operations
Mike Mirabello, Senior Graphic Artist
Susan Darbyshire, Layout Artist
Steven DeGrappo, Cover Designer
Dale Seamans, Executive Editor

Advice given is general. Readers should consult professional counsel for specific legal, ethical, or clinical questions.

Arrangements can be made for quantity discounts.

For more information, contact:

HCPro, Inc.
P.O. Box 1168
Marblehead, MA 01945
Telephone: 800/650-6787 or 781/639-1872
Fax: 781/639-2982
E-mail: *customerservice@hcpro.com*

Visit HCPro at its World Wide Web sites:
***www.hcmarketplace.com*, *www.hcpro.com*, and *www.himinfo.com*.**

11/2003
20804

Contents

About the Contributors

Angela Burnette, JD

An author and speaker, Ms. Burnette concentrates on health care regulation and complex litigation in the Atlanta law office of Alston and Bird. She advises health care providers on various aspects of risk management and has spoken on HIPAA, informed consent, and healthcare emergencies. She received a JD degree from the University of Georgia School of Law in 1993. She represents health care providers in numerous settings and has handled peer review hearings and state licensure board proceedings. She is the author of an article entitled "The Explosion of Nursing Homes Litigation and Verdicts," which was published in 1999.

Nancy Davis, MS, RHIA

Ms. Davis has worked in a variety of health care settings managing areas of health information, quality assessment, risk management, JCAHO, and safety. She has experience in both large and small health care delivery settings, including hospitals, clinics, and nursing homes. Currently, Ms. Davis is the director of privacy for Ministry Health Care, a Catholic health care system which includes a network of aligned hospitals, clinics, long-term care facilities, home care agencies and many other programs and services in Wisconsin and Minnesota. She is in charge of Ministry's HIPAA compliance program.

Cindy Ebner, MSN, RN

Ms. Ebner is the director of risk management at St. Vincent's Charity Hospital in Cleveland. She has a master's degree in nursing and has worked as a nurse legal consultant for both plaintiff and defense firms. Ms. Ebner has also taught in the undergraduate nursing programs at Case Western Reserve University in Cleveland and Walsh University in Canton, both in Ohio.

Cristine Vogel, MPH

Credited with building a culture of service at a Connecticut hospital, Ms. Vogel has more than 18 years experience in health care, currently as the manager for patient relations and advocacy at Waterbury (CT) Hospital. There, she functions as the liaison between patients and families and the hospital administration, staff and physicians to resolve complaints and facilitate service improvements. She is building a strong core of volunteer patient advocates. Ms. Vogel was the former deputy director in the State of Connecticut's Office of the Managed Care Ombudsman and a manager of market research for Aetna U.S. Healthcare.

About the Contributing Editors and Writers

Bryan Cote

Mr. Cote is an award winning writer with more than 10 years experience in health care journalism, public relations, and speech writing. As executive editor at HCPro, he researches educational training needs for health care professionals and writes and edits newsletters. In 2000, he won a *New England Press Association* award for health care feature writing and in 1999 won a *Communicator Award* for his public relations work for Charlotte Hungerford Hospital in Connecticut. Mr. Cote can be reached at *bcote@hcpro.com*.

Julie C. Pippert

Ms. Pippert has more than 10 years experience as a professional editor and writer of health care, legal, technical and business content. Ms. Pippert has worked with HCPro for many years, and has project managed and edited books such as *The Credentialing and Privileging Desk Reference* (multiple editions), *Verify and Comply* (multiple editions), *The Medical Staff Leaders' Practical Guide, Fourth Edition*, *Hugh Greeley's Answers to Common Credentialing Questions: The Comprehensive Guide*, *The JCAHO Mock Survey Made Simple*, *The Medical Executive Committee Handbook, Second Edition*, *How to Recruit and Develop Physician Leaders: A Strategy for Medical Staff Leadership Development*, *Mastering Records Completion 2: More Strategies from Medical Records Briefing*, among other projects. Ms. Pippert remains in close contact with the health care community in order to assess and address informational needs.

SECTION I

WHAT YOU NEED TO KNOW BEFORE RESPONDING TO PATIENT GRIEVANCES

SECTION I CONTENTS

Chapter 1

Responding to Patient Complaints: Legal Requirements and Issues

CHAPTER 1

Responding to Patient Complaints: Legal Requirements and Issues

Introduction: How to read this chapter and blend risk management with customer service

So you were curious. Like slowing down to see that car wreck on the freeway, you just had to have this book and read all of the mistakes your peers have made—and how they handled them. We agree. This is a critical piece of the patient relations puzzle; but it's equally important to have some legal context as you read these letters and case studies. You need to raise your expertise about how laws can shape your decisions surrounding each complaint, and how you can help your employees and management team improve the complaint management and prevention process.

In this chapter, attorney Angela Burnette has put together some sensational tips and ideas to help you do this—to blend risk management with customer service. The chapter also includes a summary of the federal and state laws that govern your work, plus a listing and analysis of those states that have recently passed laws in this area. Use this information as your guidepost. But in doing so, we urge you to weigh it against your own hospital policies, your state laws, and, to a large degree, your own view of customer service. There's no substitute for being your patients' advocate and making sure your organization keeps its promise to deliver the best service possible. After all, your patients are not only customers or clients; they are people.

Why should hospitals think about the way they handle patient complaints?

There are many good reasons why hospitals should think about how they respond to patient complaints.

First, there are federal laws that require hospitals to provide patients the opportunity to voice complaints and the right to have those complaints addressed.[1] Failure to comply with those

---

[1] *42 C.F.R. § 482.13 (Federal Conditions of Participation for hospitals participating in the Medicare or Medicaid programs) (regarding patient rights, including right to voice grievances); 45 C.F.R. §§ 160.306; 164.530 (the Health Insurance Portability and Accountability Act) (complaints regarding alleged violations of privacy rights).* See also *38 C.F.R. § 51.70(f) (right of veterans as residents of state nursing homes to voice grievances); 42 C.F.R. § 483.10(f) (right of residents in long-term care facilities to voice grievances); 42 C.F.R. § 484.10(f) (right of home health patients to voice complaints, using state telephone hotline).*

federal laws can have severe consequences, including monetary fines, civil penalties, and even possible termination from the Medicare and Medicaid programs.[2]

Second, many hospitals are accredited by the Joint Commission on Accreditation of Healthcare Organizations (JCAHO), and JCAHO has an accreditation standard that specifically deals with hospitals receiving and resolving patient complaints.[3] Failure to comply with a JCAHO standard can negatively affect a hospital's accreditation status, which could affect the hospital's reputation and standing, as well as the hospital's bottom line.

Third, some state laws require hospitals in those states to provide patients with a complaint process, some specifying the process in detail. Violation of state law could result in penalties described in the state law or, perhaps, a lawsuit based on a breach of legal duty.

But aside from legal requirements, are there other reasons to care about patient complaints? Absolutely. Patients who voiced complaints and felt the hospital listened to them and addressed those complaints may be more compliant with their treatment plans, which benefit everyone from the patient to the hospital.[4]

Plus, a hospital's resolution of complaints can mean good customer service and, in turn, good business. If patients can and do express complaints, hospitals can learn which areas may need improvement (or hospitals can learn that a particular problem still has not been adequately corrected). Patient complaints can also provide important evidence to help justify why a hospital made certain employment and medical staff decisions.[5]

Also, if a patient has complaints but does not voice them or voices the complaints but feels the hospital did not appropriately take action, the patient could then complain to friends, neighbors and coworkers. This may cost the hospital money because those people (including the unhappy patient) are more likely to choose a different hospital the next time they need health care.[6]

---

[2] See generally *42 C.F.R. §§ 488.28; 488.456; 489.53; 42 U.S.C. § 1395cc(b)(2)(B).*

[3] *Joint Commission on Accreditation of Hospitals,* Comprehensive Accreditation Manual for Hospitals: The Official Handbook, *RI.1.3.4 (2003 & CAMH Refreshed Core, Jan. 2003).*

[4] *Kathleen Doheny,* Your Body: Hospitals Are Paying More Attention to Patients' Complaints, *L.A. Times, May 15, 1990, at E2.*

[5] See Dulude v. Fletcher Allen Health Care, Inc., *807 A.2d 390 (Vt. 2002) (three patients' complaints, among other things, provided just cause for hospital's termination of nurse);* Dovin v. Beaver Dam Emergency Med., *S.C., 43 F. Supp. 2d 1027 (E.D. Wis. 1999) (in employment and alleged sexual discrimination suit, court granted summary judgment to the emergency room group employer and the hospital, based, in part, on evidence of hospital's receipt of complaints from patients and others regarding plaintiff physician's care and demeanor).*

[6] See *Teresa Dixon Murray,* Software Called Clinic's Lifesaver: System Allows Hospital to Track Patient Complaints More Efficiently, *Plain Dealer (Cleveland, Ohio) Oct. 5, 1999, at 1C (estimating a potential loss of up to $400,000 to a hospital if an unsatisfied patient later complains to 10 other individuals after discharge).*

Finally, how a hospital addresses a patient's complaint undoubtedly affects the chances a patient will later file a lawsuit against the hospital or report the problem to a government agency. For example, after years of trying to persuade a hospital to improve its interpreter services, a deaf patient ultimately resorted to filing civil rights complaints with federal agencies in order to have her complaints addressed.[7] How much time, energy, and resources (including attorneys' fees) can a hospital save by receiving and effectively resolving a patient's complaint the first time?

Let's turn now to the various legal issues facing hospitals regarding patient complaints, including what hospitals are required to do and tips for effectively receiving and resolving patient complaints.

The Medicare beneficiary complaint process: The beginning

Medicare beneficiaries (patients who receive Medicare services) have had a complaint process available to them since the late 1980s.[8] Under that process, Medicare peer review organizations (also called "PROs") generally have been required to review written complaints about the quality of services, inform the beneficiary or representative of the complaint's final disposition, and provide the involved practitioner and provider with reasonable notice and opportunity for discussion.[9]

In 1995, the Office of Inspector General (OIG) issued a report reviewing whether the Medicare beneficiary complaint process was really effective.[10] In that report, the OIG found "major flaws," including how long the whole process took to investigate and respond to complaints and the fact that Medicare beneficiaries apparently did not even know a complaint process existed.[11] Fast-forward to 2001, and the OIG issued yet another report pointing out the continuing flaws in the Medicare beneficiary complaint process.[12] In the 2001 report, the OIG commented on the utter frustration of Medicare beneficiaries, even after a peer review organization reviewed their complaints. Basically, the beneficiaries wanted, "closure after months of waiting," and they wanted to know, "what specific actions [were taken] .. in response to their particular complaints."[13]

---

[7] *Denny Walsh,* Hospital To Change Its Deaf-Patient Policies; Oroville Hospital Responds To An Angry Woman's Complaint, *Sacramento Bee, Aug. 1, 2002, at B3.*

[8] *Omnibus Budget Reconciliation Act of 1986, Pub. L. No. 99-509, 100 Stat. 1874.*

[9] *42 U.S.C. § 1320c-3(a)(14).*

[10] *Office of Inspector General, U.S. Dep't of Health and Human Services, OIE-01-93-00250, The Beneficiary Complaint Process of Medicare Peer Review Organizations (1995), available at* http://oig.hhs.gov/oei/reports/oei-01-93-00250.pdf.

[11] *Id.*

[12] *Office of Inspector General, U.S. Dep't of Health and Human Services, OIE-01-00-00060, The Medicare Beneficiary Complaint Process, A Rusty Safety Valve (2001), available at* www.hhs.gov/oig/oei/reports/oei-01-00-00060.pdf. *In that 2001 report, the OIG noted the complaint process available for Medicare beneficiaries has improved very little because (1) its accessibility is questionable (lots of busy signals when patients try to call a provided telephone number); (2) the beneficiaries did not understand the complaint process; (3) the complaint process rarely yielded in any response beyond a mere letter; and (4) the complainants did not receive a meaningful answer to their complaints.*

[13] Id. *at 12.*

In its 2001 report, the OIG recommended the Centers for Medicare and Medicaid Services (CMS, formerly the Health Care Financing Administration) provide Medicare beneficiaries with an effective complaint process. As described by the OIG, an effective complaint process instituted by CMS would: (1) be widely known and easy to use; (2) have appropriate experts, resources and methods available to assess complaints; (3) trigger appropriate interventions and monitoring based on complaints that are substantiated; (4) guide quality improvement; (5) provide regular, clear and substantive responses to complainants; (6) complete each step in the process within an established reasonable time frame, with emergent complaints handled in an expedited manner; and (7) make complaint information available to the public.[14]

Patient complaint processes now: A federal requirement for hospitals

Against this backdrop of the previously criticized Medicare patient complaint process (and some serious seclusion/restraint incidents), a new Condition of Participation was developed to provide a range of patient rights in hospitals—including, among other rights, the right to voice complaints (and the right to be free from certain seclusion/restraint methods).

When did a federal law requiring a patient complaint process come to exist? In December 1997, the Health Care Financing Administration (now CMS) issued a proposed rule to revise hospitals' Condition of Participation and to add a new Condition of Participation relating to patients' rights.[15] A Condition of Participation is a federal law listing requirements a hospital must meet in order to participate in the Medicare or Medicaid programs. In July 1999, an interim final rule was published, officially setting a new Condition of Participation dealing with patients' rights.[16] This new law, effective August 2, 1999, was, "intended to protect patient health and safety and to ensure that high quality care is provided to all patients."[17] It addressed a number of patients' rights issues, including notice, care and treatment, privacy and safety, confidentiality, certain seclusion and restraint methods and—yes—the right to voice grievances (complaints) to the hospital.[18] This federal law is referred to in these materials as, "the patients' rights Condition of Participation."

The patients' rights Condition of Participation applies to all hospitals participating in the Medicare and Medicaid programs, including short term, rehabilitation, long-term, children's, and alcohol

---

[14] Id. *at 6.*

15 xv Medicare and Medicaid Programs; Hospital Conditions of Participation; Provider Agreements and Supplier Approval, 62 Fed. Reg. 66,726 (Dec. 19, 1977) (to be codified at 42 C.F.R. pts. 416, 482, 485 and 489).

16 xvi Medicare and Medicaid Programs; Hospital Conditions of Participation: Patients' Rights, 64 Fed. Reg. 36,070 (July 2, 1999) (to be codified at 42 C.F.R. pt. 482); this interim final rule was published after a proposed revision of all hospital Conditions of Participation and addition of a new patients' rights Condition of Participation. 62 Fed. Reg. 66726.

17 xvii Medicare and Medicaid Programs; Hospital Conditions of Participation: Patients' Rights, 64 Fed. Reg. 36,070 (July 2, 1999) (to be codified at 42 C.F.R. Part 482).

18 xviii 42 C.F.R. § 482.13.

and drug facilities, as well as small rural hospitals.[19] So, all these types of hospitals must meet the requirements of the patients' rights Condition of Participation in order to participate in the Medicare and Medicaid programs, that is, in order to receive reimbursement for treating Medicare or Medicaid patients. (Note: Hospitals must meet the Medicare Conditions of Participation in order to qualify for participation in the Medicaid program.[20]) Additionally, a hospital that participates in the Medicare and Medicaid programs must meet the patients' rights Condition of Participation for all patients who receive services in that hospital—not just Medicare or Medicaid patients.[21]

TIPS

1. Hospitals should provide the notice of patients' rights as to a complaint process to both inpatients and outpatients.

2. Hospitals should provide the notice of patients' rights to all patients—whether private pay, insured, Medicaid, Medicare or other patients (such as an indigent/homeless patient who does not have Medicaid or Medicare).

Note: See Section I, Chapter 3 for best practice suggestions and sample policies and procedures.

Hospitals will be surveyed to assess whether they are meeting this Condition of Participation (including the complaint process).[22] Usually, accredited hospitals are deemed (assumed) to fulfill the Condition of Participation, so they may not be as routinely surveyed for compliance with various requirements by the state survey agencies.[23] However, regardless of their accreditation status—and even if not accredited at all—all hospitals that participate in the Medicare and Medicaid programs must comply with the Conditions of Participation. So, even if a hospital is accredited (and thus "deemed" compliant), those hospitals still must meet the requirements of the patients' rights Condition of Participation.[24] Using interpretive guidelines and survey procedures, state sur-

[19] *Medicare and Medicaid Programs; Hospital Conditions of Participation: Patients' Rights, 64 Fed. Reg. 36,070 (July 2, 1999) (to be codified at 42 C.F.R. pt. 482).* See also Hospitals Interpretive Guidelines and Survey Procedures, app. *A, Tag A 750, § 482.13 (commenting that § 482.13 (the patients' rights Condition of Participation) would not apply to "psychiatric facilities for individuals under age 21, residential treatment centers (unless these services are provided in a hospital setting) nor to "Critical Access Hospitals").*

[20] *Section 1905(a) of the Social Security Act; 42 C.F.R. § 440.10(a)(3)(iii).*

[21] See generally *Medicare and Medicaid Programs; Hospital Conditions of Participation: Quality Assessment and Performance Improvement, 68 Fed. Reg., ~~3435~~, 3437 (Jan. 24, 2003) (to be codified at 42 C.F.R. pt. 482).*

[22] *42 C.F.R. § 489.10(d); Medicare and Medicaid Programs; Hospital Conditions of Participation: Patients' Rights, 64 Fed. Reg. 36,070 (July 2, 1999) (to be codified at 42 C.F.R. pt. 482).*

[23] *Under Section 1865 of the Social Security Act, and regulations at 42 C.F.R. § 488.5.*

[24] *Centers for Medicare and Medicaid Services,* Qs/As for Hospital CoPs for Patients' Rights *(Oct. 10, 2001) available at* http://cms.hhs.gov/cop/2b1.asp.

veyors will conduct surveys to assess whether hospitals have met the patients' rights. The state survey agencies then report their recommendations to CMS.[25]

Keep in mind the patients' rights Condition of Participation is different from a "patients' bill of rights" drafted by a presidential commission in 1997–1998. In 1997, a commission appointed by President Clinton to look at health care consumers' protection and safety developed a patients' bill of rights in November 1997 with a final report in March 1998. This advisory commission listed seven rights, including the right to, "speedy complaint resolution."[26] In February 1998, President Clinton directed the Department of Health and Human Services, among others, to consider the commission's recommendations. A few of the commission's patients' "bill of rights" can also be found in the patients' rights Condition of Participation, including the reference to a complaint procedure. Remember, however, the patients' bill of rights as described by the President's commission is different than the federal law setting forth a Condition of Participation all hospitals must meet in order to participate in the Medicare and Medicaid programs.

The federal requirement for complaint processes in hospitals

Let's look now at this Condition of Participation regarding patients' rights, especially the right to voice grievances (also called complaints in this book), in more detail. Under this federal law, a hospital must

- inform each patient, or when appropriate, the patient's representative (as allowed under state law), of the patient's rights, in advance of (e.g., before) furnishing or discontinuing patient care whenever possible

- establish a process for prompt resolution of patient grievances

- inform each patient whom to contact to file a grievance

- have a governing body that approves and is responsible for the effective operation of the grievance process and this governing body must review and resolve grievances, unless it delegates the responsibility in writing to a grievance committee

- have a grievance process that includes a mechanism for the timely referral of patient concerns regarding quality of care or premature discharge to the appropriate Utilization and Quality Improvement Organization.[27]

---

[25] See generally *Medicare and Medicaid Programs; Hospital Conditions of Participation: Quality Assessment and Performance Improvement, 68 Fed. Reg. at 3,435.*

[26] *United States Department of Health & Human Services,* The Patients' Bill of Rights in Medicare and Medicaid *(Apr. 12, 1999) available at* www.hhs.gov/news/press/1999pres/990412.html.

[27] *42 C.F.R. § 482.13.*

The federal law also lists what a hospital must do, at a minimum:

- Establish a clearly explained procedure for the submission of a patient's written or verbal grievance to the hospital
- Have a grievance process that specifies the time frames for reviewing the grievance and providing a response
- Provide the patient with written notice of the hospital's decision, including
  - the name of the hospital contact person
  - the steps taken on behalf of the patient to investigate the grievance
  - the results of the grievance process
  - the date of completion[28]

For example, a hospital notifying a patient regarding the complaint process must also inform the patient that he or she can report concerns to a state survey agency, regardless of whether the patient first used the hospital's complaint process. Additionally, the hospital must provide the patient with contact information for submitting a complaint to the state survey agency (e.g., phone number and address).[29]

So, there is a federal law requiring a hospital to provide certain rights to patients, including a complaint process. Does the federal law instruct the hospital how to comply with the requirements? Not exactly. Instead, the federal government has given hospitals, "flexibility to establish policies and procedures that effectively ensure that patients and their representatives have the information necessary to exercise their rights." [30] Plus, hospitals, "need flexibility in order to keep improving how they promote patients' rights."[31] This flexibility was noted to be critical because the Condition of Participation was intended to cover "hospitals of varying sizes operating in a wide range of locations, serving diverse populations, with a variety of required notices."[32]

Hospitals have some flexibility but their policies and procedures, "will need to address how, where, and when to notify patients of the full gamut of rights to which they are entitled under the Act."[33] Despite this flexibility, hospitals want further information and clarification as to how they should give patients the rights and notice they are now required to give.

---

[28] *42 C.F.R. § 482.13(a).*

[29] *Medicare and Medicaid Programs; Hospital Conditions of Participation: Patients' Rights, 64 Fed. Reg. at 36,071.*

[30] *Medicare and Medicaid Programs; Hospital Conditions of Participation: Patients' Rights, 64 Fed. Reg. at 36,072.*

[31] Id.

[32] Id.

[33] Id.

Providing notice to patients

For example, some have questioned how and where a hospital should display the notice information about patients' rights—a display in the hospital's lobby or patient registration area, admissions packets, and/or signs in patient rooms, as well as whether all this information can be given to patients orally or in writing. One specific method approved by the government involves bundling (combining) the notice of patients' rights required under the Condition of Participation with the information hospitals already must give to patients in order to fulfill various civil rights requirements, including the Civil Rights Act of 1964, Section 504 of the Rehabilitation Act of 1973, and the Age Discrimination Act.[34] Thus, for hospitals covered by these other civil rights requirements, the notices required under the patients' rights Conditions of Participation could be effectively posted next to these already required civil rights notices.[35]

Some have asked how a hospital would provide the required notice to patients who may have problems understanding due to age, medical condition, or in an emergency. In responding to these questions, the government merely said a hospital should, "make every effort to inform the patient of his or her rights before care provision or cessation of care."[36] According to CMS, when a patient's age, condition, health or emergency situation prevents a hospital from communicating with the patient regarding his or her rights, a hospital can communicate those rights to a representative of the patient as state law permits.[37] If state law does not identify who is a patient's legal representative for particular health care decisions, then a hospital could also communicate these rights to a legal representative specifically designated by the patient, such as the agent named in a durable power of attorney for health care.[38] Even if a hospital provides notice of patient rights to a patient's representative, the hospital still should inform the patient of his rights as soon as the patient can be informed.[39] Note: Under the Health Insurance Portability and Accountability Act of 1996 (HIPAA), a hospital is permitted to communicate information to a patient's Personal Representative, a term usually defined by state law.[40] (Keep in mind HIPAA permits a hospital not to provide protected health information to a Personal Representative in certain circumstances, such as, for example, when a minor patient can obtain a health care service without parental consent or in certain abuse, neglect or endangerment situations.)[41]

---

34 Id.

35 Id.

36 *Medicare and Medicaid Programs; Hospital Conditions of Participation: Patients' Rights, 64 Fed. Reg. at 36,073.*

37 Id.

38 Id.

39 Id.

40 *45 C.F.R. § 164.502(g)(1).*

41 *45 C.F.R. § 164.502(g)(5).*

TIPS

1. The policy should delineate who, under applicable state law, would be a patient's authorized representative such that the representative would be a Personal Representative under HIPAA. (For example, depending on state law, an agent named in a patient's Durable Power of Attorney for Health Care could be a Personal Representative under HIPAA.)
2. The policy should also reference HIPAA's exceptions for Personal Representatives, as well as any applicable state laws.

Time frames for hospital response

Some have noted the patients' rights Condition of Participation did not explain how hospitals should look into patient complaints or when hospitals would be required to respond to the complaints.[42] Rather than establishing a detailed, time-specific process, the government, instead, adopted a process focused on outcome. The government noted other laws, such as state laws or even the Medicare beneficiary complaint process, might have specific time frames already in place. As to the question of time frames, the government said it expected a hospital's complaint process would "facilitate prompt, fair resolution," and "[t]he grievance process should route each concern timely to the appropriate decision-making body."[43] In sum, hospitals have "discretion" in designing and developing a process, policies and procedures on how to fulfill the patients' rights Condition of Participation, including the complaint process.[44]

Medicare patients

Additionally, we know CMS envisions "coordination" between a hospital's complaint process and the already existing referral procedures in place for Medicare beneficiaries' complaints regarding quality of care or disagreement with a coverage or discharge decision. Those Medicare beneficiaries can still contact the peer review organization to lodge a complaint. In other words, even if a

---

[42] *Medicare and Medicaid Programs; Hospital Conditions of Participation: Patients' Rights, 64 Fed. Reg. at 36,074.*

[43] Id.

[44] Id. *See also Medicare and Medicaid Programs; Hospital Conditions of Participation: Patients' Rights, 64 Fed. Reg. at 36,086 ("Regarding the grievance process, hospitals may use different approaches to effectively meet this CoP [condition of participation]. We are setting forth the general elements that should be common to grievance processes across all hospitals, but we are not explicitly delineating strategies and policies to comply with the requirement").* See generally *Medicare and Medicaid Programs; Hospital Conditions of Participation: Patients' Rights, 64 Fed. Reg. at 36,087-88 (anticipating that a hospital will provide a single "notice of patients' rights" to each patient (or representative) at the time of admission, setting forth each of the patients' rights listed in the conditions of participation. They estimate it will take approximately eight hours for a hospital to develop the required notice and will take each hospital five minutes to provide each notice).*

hospital has its own complaint process, Medicare beneficiary complaints regarding quality of care or premature discharge can and should still be referred to the peer review organization.[45]

Complaints about independent contractors and other third parties

If a patient voices a complaint regarding a physician at the hospital, the hospital should not merely tell the patient that the physician is an "independent contractor," nor should the hospital merely refer the patient to the physician's group or clinic so the patient can instead file a complaint with them.[46] Either of these statements could (incorrectly) imply to a patient 1) he/she cannot file a complaint with the hospital if it involves a physician; or 2) the hospital will not be able to investigate the complaint. Instead, the patient has the right to file a complaint with the hospital, and the hospital has the responsibility to investigate such complaint and to send a written response to the patient regarding his/her complaint.[47] This responsibility applies to patient complaints regarding non-employee physicians, as well as to patient complaints regarding other "third parties" who may be at the hospital, such as vendors, deliverymen, salesmen, etc.

Looking at the language of the patients' rights Condition of Participation, what else should a hospital do as part of its patient complaint process?

---

[45] See *Medicare and Medicaid Programs; Hospital Conditions of Participation: Patients' Rights, 64 Fed. Reg at 36,070.*

[46] See *Wisconsin Department of Health & Family Services, Bureau of Quality Assurance, June 16, 2003 memo to Wisconsin hospitals, DSL-BQA 03-010, from Jane Walters, Chief, Health Services Section via Susan Schroeder, available at* www.dhfs.state.wi.us/rl_DSL/Hospital/Hosp03010.htm.

[47] *Additionally, the hospital already has a responsibility to ensure the quality of care provided to patients by the medical staff. See id.; 42 C.F.R. § 482.12(a)(5).*

TIPS

1. A hospital's patient complaint policy should describe when the notice of patients' rights should be given to the patient or, as appropriate, the patient's "representative" (discussed later). Remember: the COP requires a hospital to provide such information before furnishing or discontinuing care whenever possible.
2. The policy should describe options for the hospital to consider in providing notice to patients with unique or special needs (such as blind or deaf patients).
3. The notice provided to patients should inform each patient whom to contact at the hospital in order to file a complaint, e.g., name, address and phone number. Remember: not all patients who file a complaint will do so while as an inpatient in the hospital—be sure to provide the complete (outside) phone number and address in case the patient wants to write or call the hospital later.
4. The hospital's complaint policy should set forth the complaint process, including how a complaint can be initiated (the hospital should consider using a complaint form), as well as the time frames (e.g., a number of days) for when a complaint will be reviewed and when the hospital will provide a response to the patient. Remember: the guidelines for how the policy is intended to work should be written as "should" and not use mandatory language such as "shall" or "must." Example: "The hospital should attempt to provide a written response to the patient within ____ days of completing the hospital's investigation, which should be within ____ days of the date when the complaint was filed."
5. The policy should address generally how the overseeing body (the governing body or the grievance committee) will review the effectiveness of the patient complaint process. For example, periodic reports could be made to the governing body or grievance committee of the number, types and resolutions of patient complaints received in a particular time period. (These reports may or may not be privileged, depending on each state's peer review laws and whether such body or committee meets the state's definition/criteria for peer review.) As another example, the governing body or grievance committee could serve as an appeal/review board if a patient is dissatisfied with the hospital's resolution of a complaint.
6. If the hospital needs to send a written response, particularly while the complaint is still under investigation, the hospital could state something similar to the following: "At this time, the hospital has not yet made a decision regarding your complaint, but is continuing to investigate the matter. We are reviewing information now and will update you. Thank you for your patience."
7. In communicating with a patient about the hospital's investigation and determination, take care not to reveal information protected by a state law privilege, such as peer review or the attorney-client privilege. A hospital should (and is obligated to) inform the patient of the results of the complaint process, but still should not reveal privileged details of the peer review process, if utilized in investigating a patient's complaint. (For example, a hospital's communication to a patient regarding a complaint should refer to facts, not conclusions.) Likewise, a hospital's response to the patient should not reveal privileged communications between the hospital and its attorney (whether in-house or outside counsel).
8. Hospitals should train their personnel—anyone who might come into contact with a patient—regarding the existence of the complaint policy. Then, if a patient voices a complaint, hospital personnel are aware of the policy and can either assist the patient in submitting the complaint or have the appropriate person come talk with the patient to facilitate filing the complaint.
9. Hospitals should try to address and resolve patient complaints filed regarding independent contractors and other third parties such as vendors or deliverymen.

What do surveyors' guidelines teach us about the hospital Conditions of Participation for patient complaints?

As with other federal requirements imposed on hospitals, "interpretive guidelines" have been issued to surveyors, so they know what information to look at when assessing a hospital's compliance during a survey. Hospital knowledge of these guidelines is crucial because the hospital will then be alert to what the agency considers important in assessing compliance. These guidelines can also provide clues or examples of what the agency would consider to be compliance with the rule.

What do these interpretive guidelines for the patients' rights Condition of Participation tell us about a hospital's patient complaint process? First, they actually define a patient grievance: "a formal, written or verbal grievance that is filed by a patient, when a patient issue cannot be resolved promptly by staff present."[48] The guidelines tell us a hospital may decide it is most effective to bundle (combine) the patients' rights and advance directive notices with the existing notices hospitals already must provide to patients, such as along with each admission packet.[49] The guidelines state a hospital "must be sensitive to the communication needs of its patients," and a hospital must present the information "in a manner and form that can be understood"; however, a hospital need not document a patient's medical record to show that it provided the patients' rights information.[50] Also, the guidelines tell us a hospital should "have a process to implement a relatively minor change in a more timely manner than a written response"—for example, this means a hospital should be able to remedy a housekeeping matter quickly without having to wait until the hospital formulates and sends a written response.[51] The interpretive guidelines also remind us surveyors will speak with staff, patients and families to assess whether they know about and are familiar with the grievance process and patients' rights.

What tips can we learn from the interpretive guidelines regarding a hospital's grievance process for patients?

---

[48] Hospitals Interpretive Guidelines and Survey Procedures, *app. A, Tag A 752, § 482.13, at A-172.*

[49] Hospitals Interpretive Guidelines and Survey Procedures, *app. A, Tag A 751, § 482.13, at A-171.*

[50] Id. *at Tag A 751, § 482.13, A-171.*

[51] Id. *at Tag A 752, § 482.13, A-172.*

TIPS

1. When communicating patients' rights, including the right to voice complaints, the hospital should comply with civil rights laws by providing interpretation for certain non-English speaking individuals, assistance to deaf or blind patients, and provide other communication assistance such as using large print materials, signs, magnifying glass, Braille, or sign language.
2. Hospital staff should be aware of and know what options are available if a patient has special communication needs, but wants to file a complaint. (For example, a hospital could offer assistance to a patient who is not able to or would otherwise have difficulty completing a hospital's complaint form, such as a patient recovering from a stroke.)
3. When informing a patient (or patient's representative, as appropriate) about his or her rights, the hospital should
   - inform the patient he or she can submit a complaint directly to the state agency, regardless of whether the patient also used the hospital's complaint process first
   - provide the patient with such state agency's contact information, such as phone number and address
4. If a Medicare patient also requests review by a PRO, the hospital should promptly forward the request to the PRO. (If the Medicare beneficiary has also filed a complaint with the hospital, the hospital should still investigate and report the hospital's response to the patient.)
5. Hospital staff should be aware of the hospital's complaint policy, understand it applies to both oral and written complaints, and know the process for submitting a patient complaint.
6. A hospital's complaint policy should encourage all personnel to alert the appropriate hospital staff regarding any patient grievance. Although the policy should specify guidelines or time frames for a hospital's response, the hospital should have a mechanism by which a relatively minor matter (such as bedding) can be resolved quickly. (Note: Even if a minor matter is resolved quickly and orally communicated to the patient, the hospital should still send a written response to the patient.)
7. Likewise, a hospital's policy should provide for immediate review of grievances posing a possible patient danger, such as abuse or neglect.
8. Staff should try to resolve promptly issues or concerns voiced by patients. If such resolution is not possible or appropriate, the patient should be reminded of his or her right to file a complaint. (Note by the author: If a patient declines to file a complaint, but the matter is serious or the patient is quite unhappy, a hospital might consider documenting that the patient was advised of his right to file a complaint, but chose not to do so. This documentation could be made, for example, on an incident report form or otherwise provided to risk management.)
9. Whether a grievance is minor or serious, the hospital should look to the "substance" of the problem and identify, investigate and resolve any "deeper or systemic" issues brought to light by the grievance. (For example, is bedding an issue because, perhaps, the temperature used for hot water in the laundry is not sufficiently high? Look at the hot water temperature to help get to the root of the identified problem. Document the steps taken by the hospital to investigate the complaint.)
10. After investigating the grievance and determining the hospital's assessment and response, the hospital should provide a written response to the patient or patient's representative of the hospital's response/resolution in a way the patient or representative will understand. This could include, but is not limited to, actually meeting with the patient or family as appropriate.
11. The hospital should seek to learn from the complaints and incorporate and apply this education as part of its continuing quality improvement/peer review efforts. For example, a QA, QI or peer review committee could review and analyze how the grievance process is working, e.g., identifying trends and providing "oversight" to the process. (If the hospital or this committee identifies steps the hospital can and should take to prevent a complaint from happening again, "follow through" by taking (and documenting) those corrective measures.)
12. The review and analysis of the hospital's grievance process—whether by the governing body or another committee—should be reflected in the minutes of such entity's meetings.

A new complaints database

In August 2003, CMS published a notice regarding a new tracking system for complaints and incidents.[52] This program is called "ASPEN Complaints/Incidents Tracking System" or "ACTS." The system is designed to "track and process complaints and incidents reported against Medicare/Medicaid/CLIA providers and suppliers and to maintain information on laboratory directors and owners."[53] CMS developed the ACTS system to better track patient complaints, partially in response to the criticisms previously voiced regarding the federal government's handling of investigating and responding to patient complaints.

The ACTS system seeks to enhance efficiency by allowing collection of federal and state information in one database rather than multiple systems.[54] It allows CMS to track and manage complaints from intake through to investigation and final disposition. The ACTS system will track a broad range of complaint data in categories such as complainants, witnesses, residents/patient information, survey team members, alleged perpetrators and others.[55]

Importantly, CMS will use this database information to assist in the survey and certification process of Medicare/Medicaid/CLIA providers, assist state agencies in assessing the quality of provider and suppliers services, support litigation and research involving the agency, and help administer state and federal programs, among other things.[56]

The August 2003 notice outlines in detail the proposed "routine uses" (and the criteria and restrictions for such uses) by CMS of the information in the database, including certain disclosures to the Department of Justice, CMS employees or contractors, a Quality Improvement Organization, certain state agencies (including Medicaid agencies), the Office of Inspector General, to a national accreditation organization with deeming authority (such as JCAHO), and to certain law enforcement, among others.[57] CMS proposes to prohibit release of even non-identifying data to entities other than those listed under "routine uses" in the notice, if "there is a possibility that an individual can be identified through implicit deduction based on small cell sizes."[58]

Although the actual effect of the ACTS system remains to be seen, it is certainly fair to say hospitals should expect to see a more organized, efficient and coordinated effort by CMS towards patient complaints.

---

[52] *HHS Centers for Medicare & Medicaid Services; Privacy Act of 1974; Report of New System, 68 Fed. Reg. 50795 (Aug. 22, 2003).*
[53] *Id. "CLIA" refers to the Clinical Laboratory Improvement Amendments of 1988.*
[54] *Id.*
[55] *Id. at 50797.*
[56] *Id. at 50795-50796.*
[57] *Id. at 50798-50799.*
[58] *Id. at 50798.*

JCAHO accreditation standard regarding patient complaints

JCAHO has an accreditation standard in place specifically governing patient complaints.[59] (Note: please see the text in this endnote for important information about JCAHO's 2004 pre-publication standard regarding patient complaints.) Under the current accreditation standard, which is a "Patient Rights" standard, a hospital should "demonstrate respect" for a patient's needs for "resolution of complaints."[60] JCAHO's "Intent" for this standard is for the hospital to have "a way of providing" for a patient's right to "voice complaints about his or her care, and to have those complaints reviewed and, when possible, resolved."[61]

JCAHO provides an example of how hospitals could implement this patient complaint standard:

> The hospital has a formal process for reviewing patient complaints and helping to resolve conflicts. This process includes a plan to inform patients and their families of their right to make complaints and how to go about having them resolved. This process also involves a patient advocate or representative who reviews the complaint and consults with the appropriate hospital staff (for example, nursing, medical staff, housekeeping). Those issues that cannot be resolved in this manner are referred to the hospital administration for intervention.[62]

Although this accreditation standard sounds relatively general, it is still important to look at it line by line and think about how a hospital should consider documenting its compliance for surveyors. Having a formal process in all likelihood, means having a written policy and procedure for receiving, addressing and resolving patient complaints.

---

59 *Joint Commission on Accreditation of Healthcare Organizations,* Comprehensive Accreditation Manual for Hospitals: The Official Handbook, *at RI.1.3.4. Note the numbering for this JCAHO standard will change in 2004, to become RI.2.120. Based on the 2004 pre-publication JCAHO standards, the new RI.2.120 will state, "The organization addresses the resolution of complaints from patients and their families." See* www.jcaho.org/accredited+organizations/hospitals/standards/new+standards/2004+standards.htm. *Based on the JCAHO's 2004 pre-publication materials, the "elements of performance" for this patient complaint standard will be as follows: "1. The organization informs patients, families, and staff about the complaint resolution process; 2. The organization receives, reviews, and, when possible, resolves complaints from patients and their families; 3. The organization responds to individuals making a significant (as defined by the organization) or recurring complaint; 4. The organization informs patients about their right to file a complaint with the state authority; and 5. Patients can freely voice complaints and recommend changes without being subject to coercion, discrimination, reprisal, or unreasonable interruption of care, treatment, and services." Id. This chapter does not analyze JCAHO's pre-publication standards for patient complaints, but note, for example, JCAHO's pre-publication standard would have a hospital provide a response when a patient makes a "significant" or "recurring" complaint, while the Federal Hospital Condition of Participation for patients' rights, 42 C.F.R. § 482.13(a)(2), requires a hospital to provide written notice of its decision to patients who file a complaint (e.g., all complaints—not just significant or recurring ones).*

60 *Joint Commission on Accreditation of Healthcare Organizations,* Comprehensive Accreditation Manual for Hospitals: The Official Handbook, *at RI.1.3.4.*

61 Id. *at RI-15.*

62 Id. *at RI-16.*

Having a plan to inform patients involves thinking about when such information should be given to patients, in what format, and how to do so when patients are unconscious or in an emergency condition. Also, whether to inform patients' families about their right to make complaints also means considering the patients' privacy rights and not disclosing information to the families in violation of state or federal privacy laws. Using a patient advocate or representative would involve the hospital dedicating (and training) a particular person or department to receive the complaints, talking with the patient, and consulting the appropriate staff at the hospital to resolve the complaints. Finally, referral of unresolved complaints to hospital administration for intervention means thinking about who in hospital administration should receive this information, what is meant by intervention and what should occur if complaints are still unresolved after such intervention.

Although the JCAHO standard is somewhat broad, a hospital can take some steps to fit within JCAHO's description of a complaint process.

TIPS

1. Address when and how a hospital should provide such information in instances where a patient is unconscious or in an emergency condition.

2. Address when and how the hospital might look to providing such information to a patient's family rather than the patient—while still complying with state and federal privacy laws.

3. Designate and train a hospital representative (or representatives) to receive the complaints and talk with the patients or family (if appropriate).

4. Identify who such representative can contact in each hospital department to discuss (and hopefully resolve) a patient's complaint regarding that department.

5. Consider having the policy address at what point a complaint remains "unresolved."

6. Identify who at the hospital administration level will receive and review unresolved complaints.

7. Specify some examples of "intervention" steps administration can take. (It is impossible for a policy to list all such examples, especially when patient complaints will differ and might be handled best on a case-by-case basis. So, for example, a policy could state something to the following effect: Administration should review unresolved patient complaints and consider intervention options, including but not limited to, contacting the patient, discussing the matter with the appropriate department head, and/or referring the matter to a peer review committee if appropriate. It is impossible for this policy to identify the entire range of intervention options, as each patient complaint will be different. However, the hospital will strive to enable patients to voice complaints and to have such complaints reviewed and, if possible, resolved.)

Individual state laws regarding patient complaints

This chapter, up to this point, has reviewed the federal patients' rights Condition of Participation, and the national accreditation standards regarding patient complaint procedures. However, there are also laws at the individual state level, which also deal with a hospital's complaint process for patients.

Several states have enacted laws specifically requiring patient complaint procedures. Some of these state laws apply to "hospitals."[63] For example, Maryland, Massachusetts, New Jersey, and New York each have laws addressing patients' right to complain and/or a hospital's complaint procedure.[64] Other state laws, such as in New Jersey, govern "health care facilities" and specifically require those facilities to provide patients with certain notices regarding patient rights, including the right to file or submit a complaint.[65]

---

[63] See e.g., *Md. Code Ann., Health-Gen. § 19-309 (investigation of complaints in hospitals and residential treatment centers; issues relating to the practice of medicine or licensure conduct of a health professional shall be referred to the hospital for resolution. If the Department finds the hospital or center has not satisfactorily addressed the complaint, or where the complaint alleges the existence of a life-threatening deficiency, the Department shall conduct an independent investigation.)* See generally *Md. Code Ann., Health-Gen. § 19-319(g)(2)(iv) (minimum standards for a risk management program shall include "a formal written program for addressing patient complaints;" the hospital's risk management program is a condition of licensure); Mass. Regs. Code tit. 105, § 103.330 (requiring hospitals to develop written procedures to assure "prompt and complete investigations of all serious complaints which are filed against employees of the hospital or members of its medical staff;" at a minimum, the procedure must include designation of a senior hospital administration member; establishment of a reporting procedure which assures that designated administrator will receive written reports of serious complaints within one day from hospital staff; development by the designated administrator of a written investigation process, which shall include minimum elements set forth in more detail on the regulation, and requiring complaint files to be made available for inspection by agents of the Department of Public Health).* See also *N.J. Admin. Code tit. 8, § 43g-5.2(g) (requiring administrative and hospital-wide policies and procedures as hospital licensing standards, including "a complaint procedure for patients, families, and other visitors. The procedure shall include, at least, a system for receiving complaints, a specified response time, assurance that complaints are referred appropriately for review, development of resolutions, and follow-up action.); N.Y. Comp. Codes R. & Regs. tit. 10, § 405.7 (patients' rights; hospitals) (requiring that hospitals provide patients or patient representatives with copies of their rights at the time of admission, and, for outpatients and emergency patients, provided to the patient and/or his or her representative, and also posted in clearly viewed areas of the hospital, such rights to include the right to "register complaints and recommend changes in policies and services to the facility's staff, the governing authority and in the New York State Department of Health without fear of reprisal;" and "express complaints about the care and services provided and to have the hospital investigate such complaints." Id. at ¶¶ 22-23). Under this New York law, the hospital "shall provide the patient or his/her designee with a written response if requested by the patient indicating the findings of the investigation. The hospital shall notify the patient or his/her designee that if the patient is not satisfied with the hospital's oral or written response, the patient may complain to the New York State Department of Health's Office of Health Systems Management. The hospital shall provide the telephone number of the local area office of the Health Department to the patient.")*

[64] Id.

[65] See, e.g., *N.J. Stat. Ann. § 26:2H-12.7 (Health Care Facilities Planning Act) (stating a patient may file a written complaint against a hospital for failure to comply with provisions of this bill, or any rule or regulation adopted pursuant to this bill, either with the hospital or with the Department of Health. The hospital or Department of Health shall respond promptly in writing to the complaint, and the Department of Health shall investigate a written complaint and report its findings to the hospital and the patient).*

Some state laws, such as the one in Virginia, contain detailed requirements for handling patient complaints, even setting forth required written notifications and timelines, as well as documentation requirements.[66] Other state patient complaint laws, such as those in Georgia, Illinois, Maryland and Hawaii, specifically apply to a particular type of health care facility or health care provider, like mental health, extended care or home health.[67]

Hospitals and health care facilities need to be aware of their state's laws regarding complaint procedures and need to make sure policies and procedures are consistent with these state law requirements, some of which are quite detailed. These hospitals may wish to have their local counsel review their hospital policies to ensure they are consistent with these state laws.

Responding to patient complaints: Potential issues regarding admissions of liability

We know hospitals are supposed to respond to patient complaints by communicating with the patient about his or her complaint and the action, if any, taken by the hospital. In responding to a patient's complaint—whether responding orally or in writing—hospitals should be aware of potential legal issues, including whether the hospital's "response" could later be used as evidence against the hospital.

Therefore, hospitals should know some general principles about "admissions," offers to compromise or settle, and offers of benevolence or sympathy. Additionally, hospitals in certain states

---

[66] See, e.g., *12 Va. Admin. Code § 5-408-180 (Virginia regulation governing hospitals, nursing homes, and related institutions and services, setting forth detailed system for resolution of complaints brought by covered persons or providers acting on behalf of a covered person and with a covered person's consent, including complaints regarding availability, delivery, quality of health care services, or any other matter pertaining to the covered person's contractual relationship or status as a third party beneficiary). This Virginia law requires written notification to covered persons of the procedure, including telephone numbers and addresses, a description of the process used to investigate and resolve the complaints, including specific timeframes, and information regarding how the process will be used to document and track the status of all complaints). Timeframes for responding to complaints must take into account clinical urgency but shall not exceed 30 days from the receipt of the complaint, and the complaint must be resolved within 60 days of the date the complaint was received. The Virginia licensee must keep complaint records, including using a complaint identifier and tracking the date the complaint was received, a general description for the reason for the complaint, the date of each review and hearing, if any, the number of days to gather the information necessary to resolve the complaint, the date the complaint was closed, how the complaint was resolved, the record of internal actions which were necessary as a result of the resolution, and notification to the covered person of the resolution. Id. Such complaint records must be maintained from the date of the licensee's last examination and for no less than five years. Id.*

[67] See, e.g., *O.C.G.A. § 37-3-149 (requiring mental health facilities in Georgia to establish procedures where "complaints of the patient or complaints of the staff concerning treatment of the patient can be speedily heard, with final decisions to be made by the superintendent, the regional state hospital administrator, or an advisory committee, whichever is appropriate. ... However, the patient shall not be required to utilize these procedures in lieu of other available legal remedies"); 210 Ill. Comp. Stat. 87/15 (Requiring health facilities to instruct patients to direct complaints regarding interpreter services to the Illinois Department of Public Health) (note: see recent amendment (new section 16), effective January 1, 2004, regarding patient complaints to Department); Md. Regs. Code tit. 10, § 07.09.16 (setting forth detailed complaint procedure for extended care facilities and comprehensive care facilities); Haw. Rev. Stat. §334E-2 (discussing mental health client's right to a grievance procedure).*

should learn and take advantage of the protection those states offer to statements of apologies, expressions of regret or sympathy. Finally, all hospitals—no matter where they are located—should know about "cooperation clauses" in their insurance policies and whether certain statements by the hospital could violate a cooperation clause and possibly lead an insurer to fight or deny coverage for a particular incident.

Admissions generally

A hospital's written statement to a patient, payer or other person (including a patient's attorney) admitting liability for a patient's incident or complication could have far-reaching consequences. For example, the person who receives a copy of such a written letter could institute a lawsuit, forward the statement to a newspaper, or send the statement to government payers, such as Medicare/Medicaid, which paid for services the hospital may have admittedly provided negligently or otherwise improperly.

For purposes of evidence at trial, a court could admit the hospital's written statement as what is called an "admission against interest." Generally, for a statement to constitute an admission of liability against a party to a lawsuit, the statement must be made by a party or an agent or employee of the party.[68] However, the statements or admissions of some agents or employees may not legally bind the hospital if they did not have authority to bind the hospital.[69]

So, if an unhappy or injured patient later files a lawsuit arising from a particular incident at a hospital, and if the hospital previously wrote the patient a letter admitting the incident was the hospital's fault, the hospital's written statement might be used as evidence against the hospital at trial. If the hospital had already admitted responsibility for the incident, a judge might find the jury only has to decide damages (how much money the hospital should pay) because the issue of who is responsible has already been decided. That type of decision by the judge may adversely affect a hospital's ability to 1) present expert evidence showing the incident can arise in the absence of negligence; 2) present evidence as to the standard of care; 3) present evidence of contributory-comparative negligence by the patient or others; or 4) present information later learned by the hospital showing the incident complained of was actually not the hospital's fault.

---

[68] See, *for example, O.C.G.A. § 24-3-33 (admissions by agents); § 24-3-34 (admissions by parties) (both Georgia laws).*

[69] See e.g., HCP III Woodstock, Inc. v. Healthcare Services Group, Inc., *254 Ga. App. 242, 562 S.E.2d 255 (2002) (an employee's statement, made 13 days after a fire in a nursing home, that he had seen and reported a dryer emitting flames prior to the fire was not admissible as an omission of a party opponent, because as a mere employee he did not have authority to bind the provider, and, since 13 days had passed since the fire, the statement was not made contemporaneously).*

Furthermore, a written statement by the hospital admitting liability could be used against a hospital in later lawsuits—even those not involving the original incident or patient. For example, a plaintiff's lawyer might contend a written statement admitting liability shows the hospital previously knew about a particular problem, but did not correct it. Thus, the lawyer might try to use a hospital's written statement admitting liability as the basis for what are generally known as "punitive damages" against the hospital in a later lawsuit arising from the same (now known but uncorrected) problem. These types of damages are called "punitive" because they are intended to punish a wrongdoer who had prior notice of a problem but chose not to fix it; these damages are in addition to the other types of money damages (such as lost wages or medical expenses) that might be awarded to a patient.

Special circumstances regarding some admissions

Not all statements, even if made, may be admitted as evidence in a later lawsuit. Some states have laws which specifically protect certain statements from later being admissible evidence, and courts have refused to admit evidence of such comments (including even an offer to pay or reduce medical expenses) if 1) such offer is an impulsive act of benevolence and sympathy; or 2) if such offer was made with a view to compromise (or settle) the matter. So, if a hospital's verbal or written statement to a patient is impulsively made out of sympathy or made to settle a dispute, there is a greater chance a judge would not admit the hospital's statement into evidence against the hospital, depending, of course, on the scope and exceptions set forth in each particular state's laws. Statements made out of sympathy or in an effort to settle are discussed in more detail below.

Admissions resulting from silence

Keep in mind another set of laws may also come into play. For example, evidence of a hospital not responding to a patient's letter might be used against a hospital in a later lawsuit. Under this evidence rule, where parties are engaged in a business or other type of relationship where it is unlikely an untrue communication would be ignored, then the failure to send a reply letter can be evidence of an "admission" by reason of silence—if the complaining letter contained statements which the recipient would normally deny if untrue.[70] (In other words, would it be reasonable for the letter's author to expect the letter's recipient to reply and correct what the letter says?) For example, in one case, a patient developed an infection after cortisone injections. The patient's husband sent a letter to the physician, complaining and asking him to reimburse them for the medical expenses incurred because of the infection. At trial, the judge admitted the husband's letter into evidence. On appeal, the court held the trial judge properly admitted the letter into evidence because the physician had an "on-going relationship with [the patient and her husband] at the time the letter was sent, and it would be improbable that a physician would ignore a letter

[70] See Crain v. Allison, *443 A.2d 558 (D.C. 1982).*

placing on him liability for an infection which he did not cause."[71] Therefore, hospitals should carefully review letters from disgruntled patients, family members and even payers—taking care to respond to (and deny, if appropriate) facts contained in those letters that are untrue or inaccurate—otherwise, a non-responding hospital may face an uphill battle arguing it did not admit such facts by remaining silent.

Admitting liability? A novel approach

Despite these concerns about making admissions, some hospitals have chosen to proceed by making candid admissions to patients/families after an incident. (Note: JCAHO has a standard requiring a responsible licensed independent practitioner or his or her designee to inform patients and their families, when appropriate, regarding "unanticipated outcomes."[72]) Consistent with the results of some studies regarding malpractice litigation (e.g., that it is not always quality of care and negligence which motivates patients to file suit),[73] some hospitals are trying a new way to handle medical errors (and communicate them to patients and families). For example, the Veteran's Administration Hospital in Lexington, Kentucky reportedly handles medical errors by candidly talking with the patient or family about the event and informing the patient or family of their right to file suit.[74] The Lexington VA Hospital has apparently continued handling such incidents in this manner "because administration and staff believe that it is the right thing to do and because it has resulted in unanticipated financial benefits...."[75]

A hospital may want to consider using this somewhat novel approach in certain circumstances. Such proactive discussions with patients and families may benefit a hospital by 1) reducing attorney fees and expenses that a hospital would otherwise incur from lengthy litigation; 2) resulting in early, and often lower, settlements with the patient or family; 3) avoiding exposure to punitive damages (which can be a big risk at trial in some cases) by resolving the matter early; and 4)

---

[71] Id. *at 565.*

[72] *Joint Commission on Accreditation of Healthcare Organizations,* Comprehensive Accreditation Manual for Hospitals: The Official Handbook, *at RI.1.2.2. Based on the 2004 pre-publication JCAHO standards, the new RI.1.2.2 will be renumbered as RI.2.90 and will state, "Patients and, when appropriate, their families are informed about the outcomes of care, treatment, and services, including unanticipated outcomes."* See www.jcaho.org/accredited+organizations/hospitals/standards/new+standards/2004+standards.htm. *Based on JCAHO's pre-publication materials, the "Elements for Performance" for the new RI.290 are as follows: "At a minimum, the patient and when appropriate, his or her family, is informed about the following: 1. Outcomes of care, treatment and services that have been provided that the patient (or family) must be knowledgeable about to participate in current and future decisions affecting the patient's care, treatment, and services; 2. Unanticipated outcomes of care, treatment, and services that relate to sentinel events considered reviewable by the Joint Commission; and 3. The responsible LIP or his or her designee informs the patient (and when appropriate, his or her family) about those unanticipated outcomes of care, treatment, and services) see Element of Performance 2 [above])." Id. (Note: "LIP" refers to an licensed independent practitioner). Per JCAHO, "in settings where there is no LIP, the staff member responsible for the care of the patient is responsible for sharing information about such outcomes." Id.*

[73] *Wendy Levinson,* Physician-Patient Communication: A Key to Malpractice Prevention, *272 JAMA 1619 (1994), citing S.S. Entman, et al.,* The Relationship Between Malpractice Claims History and Subsequent Obstetric Care, *272 JAMA 1588 (1994).*

[74] See *S.S. Kraman and G. Hamm, Risk Management: Extreme Honesty May Be The Best Policy, 131 Annals of Internal Medicine 963 (1999).*

[75] *Id. at 964.*

negating a later allegation that the hospital committed fraud by "covering up" the incident (in other words, a candid disclosure of the incident likely begins the statute of limitations). Additionally, such proactive discussions ultimately may improve hospital-patient relations and the hospital's community image.

There is no absolute rule about whether a hospital should admit to a patient or family that the hospital made an "error" or "mistake." It may be too early for a hospital to know what really happened regarding a patient's complaint, and such statements could be viewed as an admission of liability. Furthermore, a hospital's admission of an "error" or "mistake" might lead some patients or families to file suit who otherwise would not have done so. With some patient complaints, however, some hospitals might decide it is best to fully admit to an error. If a hospital is considering whether to proceed down this road, however, there are some important issues to evaluate. The following nine crucial tips outline these.

Figure 1.1

Issues to Think about when Considering Whether to Openly Admit Liability

1. Assess whether an "error" really happened and be sure. While the patient is still hospitalized, the hospital may believe (but may not actually know) what truly happened. Two weeks later, the hospital may discover the incident was not really an error, or discover that an error occurred but it was the fault of a person or entity other than the hospital.

2. Determine whether the "error" was actually the proximate cause of any harm. For example, a hospital could have made a mistake, but it did not cause any harm or was unrelated to the harm that occurred.

3. Evaluate whether everyone at the hospital agrees with making an admission. The hospital should not respond to a patient complaint by making an admission, if others involved in the patient's care are still disagreeing about what happened.

4. Assess the chance a lawsuit would be filed by the patient or family. Many hospitals handle such conversations under the assumption a lawsuit will be filed.

5. Identify the best person to deliver the news to the patient or family. (Sometimes, the treating physician may not be the best person to talk with the family, due to the physician's demeanor or, perhaps, his or her inability to accept and admit responsibility.)

6. The hospital should consider adopting a written policy describing who can attend such a meeting between the hospital and the patient or family. For example, a hospital may want consider having a chaplain present.

7. Before making an admission, the hospital should talk with its insurance company regarding any "cooperation" or anti-admission clauses in the hospital's insurance policy. These clauses may affect whether an insurance company later tries to deny coverage for an incident, as discussed later in this chapter.

8. If the decision has been made to admit an error, consider communicating such admissions out of benevolence/sympathy or as an attempt to negotiate a settlement or compromise of the dispute (discussed below) in order to help protect such statements from later being admitted as evidence.

9. If the decision has been made to admit an error, take care not to waive or disclose peer review privileged information (or attorney-client privileged information).

Note: See Chapter 7, "Follow-up replies: Responding throughout the process and communicating the status of the investigation" for a sample of a letter that admits liability. The section is titled, "Issue: Iatrogenic injury discovered after discharge."

Voluntary offers of benevolence or sympathy

Overview

Generally, actions that constitute a voluntary offer of assistance "made on the impulse of benevolence or sympathy" should be "encouraged" and should not be considered admissions of liability.[76] Stated another way, courts are hesitant to admit into evidence voluntary payments that are made for "humanitarian purposes." Whether a hospital's offer to pay or reduce medical expenses is actually an act of benevolence and sympathy, however, depends on the particular facts and circumstances at issue.

At least some courts appear to favor finding acts of benevolence rather than admissions of liability. For example, in one case, the hospital's payment of lost wages and medical expenses to a patient with financial difficulties (so the patient could buy Christmas presents for her children) was deemed an act of benevolence and sympathy, rather than an admission.[77] In another (older) case, a lawsuit was filed against a physician, alleging he negligently removed two permanent teeth during a child's tonsillectomy.[78] Soon after the operation, the physician apparently offered the patient's father a check for $300 to use toward the child's resulting dental bill. At trial, the court held the offering of a check was not an admission of liability, because the offer was "inspired by motives of friendship and human kindness," particularly because the physician was a neighbor and (formerly) good friends with the child and her parents.[79] (It is much more common, however, for these types of potential "benevolence" cases to involve statements made by drivers after automobile accidents.[80])

---

[76] Deese v. Carroll City County Hosp., *203 Ga. App. 148, 150, 416 S.E.2d 127, 129 (1992); Widner v. Brookins, Inc., 236 Ga. App. 563, 512 S.E.2d 405 (1999).* See also Novick v. Dillon, *44 Va. Cir. 111, 112 (1997) (holding doctor's alleged offer to pay hospital bills the day after surgery was inadmissible, finding that offers to pay an injured party's medical bills, "whether made out of a sense of religious or moral obligation, sympathy, conscience, or anything else, should be encouraged" and thus are not admissible as evidence of liability unless they contain an express admission of liability).* See generally, Phinney v. Vinson, *605 A.2d 849 (Vt. 1992) (finding a physician's alleged apology for his failure to perform a procedure adequately, while potentially admissible, was not sufficient to establish a standard of care or the breach thereof);* Senesac v. Assocs. in Obstetrics and Gynecology, *449 A.2d 900 (Vt. 1982) (finding doctor's admission of a mistake did not necessarily show a deviation from the appropriate standard of care, but rather expressed the physician's belief her performance did not meet her own standards of care and skill);* Locke v. Pachtman, *521 N.W.2d 786, 789 (Mich. 1994) (surgeon's alleged statement that "I knew the needle was too small when I used it" did not establish the standard of care and breach of that standard); Zolk v. Simon, 44 Pa. D. & C. 3d 533 (1997) (without expert testimony establishing a breach of the applicable standard of care, a physician's alleged statement that he made a mistake when he damaged a nerve was insufficient to establish negligence). For details as to standard of care issues raised by a physician's admissions of negligence, see David M. Epstein, Annotation,* Medical Malpractice: Physician's Admission of Negligence as Establishing Standard of Care and Breach of That Standard, *42 A.L.R. 5th 1 (1996).*

[77] Deese, *203 Ga. App. at 150, 416 S.E.2d at 129.*

[78] Fields v. Rutledge, *284 S.W.2d 659 (Ky. Ct. App. 1955).*

[79] Fields, *284 S.W.2d at 662.*

[80] See e.g., *in Georgia,* Neubert v. Vigh, *218 Ga. App. 693, 462 S.E.2d 808 (1995) (in accident case, offer by driver's parent to pay victim's medical expenses/insurance deductibles was motivated by benevolence and sympathy due to financial difficulties of victim);* Rosequist v. Pratt, *201 Ga. App. 45, 410 S.E.2d 316, 317 (1991) (in accident case, motorist's offer to "take care of medical and funeral expenses" for child was not admission but was instead a voluntary offer of assistance based on sympathy);* Steverson v. Eason, *194 Ga. App. 273, 390 S.E.2d 424 (1990) (in accident case, driver's statement after accident he felt responsible and would do whatever he could for the plaintiff was an expression of benevolence or sympathy);* Evans v. Batchelor, *137 Ga. App. 629, 224 S.E.2d 752 (1976) (driver's statements after accident expressing regret and stating his insurance would take care of everything were not admissions of liability).*

If a hospital wishes to write off or reduce a patient's bill, a stronger argument might exist that the hospital was motivated by benevolence or sympathy if such offer was 1) made at or very soon after the incident; 2) in response to the plaintiff's financial difficulties; 3) by someone who was not involved in causing the injury; and 4) in cases where the defendant has very little to no potential liability. Additionally, if the hospital voluntarily reduces a patient's bill for injuries due to acts of third parties or independent contractors (over whom the hospital may not have control), one can argue the hospital's actions were more likely expressions of benevolence rather than admissions of liability. In cases where the hospital chooses to write off or reduce a patient's bill for benevolent purposes, the hospital can take certain steps to show such actions were motivated by kind intentions, rather than an admission of liability.

TIPS

1. The hospital should document internally the reason(s) for the write-off or reduction, e.g., a patient's financial problems or a difficult personal situation involving the patient or family (example: a fire destroying their home).

2. Any correspondence to the patient regarding the write-off should state the same reasons. The internal documentation and correspondence regarding this write-off would not discuss the hospital's potential liability, since the hospital is acting benevolently by writing off some of the bill, even though it does not have liability. For example, a letter to the patient could specifically refer to the hospital's sympathy for the patient's situation, such as the recent loss of her home due to a tornado, a recent layoff, etc.

3. In certain cases, however, where the hospital may have some liability (e.g., retained sponges and incorrect medication) the hospital may wish to pursue compromise or settlement of the claim.

New State Laws Protecting Apologies

Several states have enacted statutes providing that certain types of apologies or expressions of sympathy made after an accident occurs are inadmissible to show liability. Massachusetts was the first state to do so in 1986—a state legislator introduced the bill after a person responsible for the death of his daughter did not apologize for fear of the apology being used against him in litigation.[81] The Massachusetts statute provides that statements or gestures expressing sympathy or general sense of benevolence are inadmissible as evidence of admission of liability.[82]

[81] See *Jonathan R. Cohen,* Legislating Apology: The Pros and Cons, *70 U. Cin. L. Rev. 819, 828 (2002).*

[82] *Mass. Gen. Laws ch. 233, § 23D.*

California, Florida, Texas, and Washington have also enacted laws stating an apology or expression of sympathy after an accident is not evidence of an admission of liability, but statements of fault are still admissible.[83]

Interestingly, Oregon and Colorado passed laws in 2003 that are even broader in scope. Under Oregon's new law, "any expression of regret or apology ... including an expression ... that is made in writing, orally or by conduct, does not constitute an admission of liability for any purpose."[84] Also, anyone "who is licensed by the Board of Medical Examiner, or any other person who makes an expression of regret or apology on behalf of a person who is licensed by the Board of Medical Examiners" cannot have their deposition taken in any civil or administrative proceeding, including arbitration or mediation, regarding such expression of regret or apology (including expressions made in writing, orally or by conduct).[85] This is good news for Oregon hospitals, physicians, and physicians' employees, although some might contend the law could have been written even more broadly. (For example, the Oregon law specifically prevents "depositions," but one could argue the Oregon law may not completely block other discovery methods generally available to obtain information during a lawsuit, such as interrogatories, request for production of documents, request for admissions, and even live testimony at trial.)

Colorado's new law goes a bit further than Oregon's, specifically excluding statements admitting fault as well those expressing sympathy or benevolence.[86] Generally, under this new law, if all the criteria listed below are met, the following statements and conduct are no longer admissible as evidence to show liability or to show an admission against interest:

- Any and all statements, affirmations, gestures, or conduct which expresses apology, fault, sympathy, commiseration, condolence, compassion, or a general sense of benevolence

- Which are made by a health care provider or an employee of a health care provider to the alleged victim, a relative of the alleged victim, or a representative of the alleged victim

- Which relate to the discomfort, pain, suffering, injury, or death of the alleged victim

- Made as the result of the unanticipated outcome of medical care[87]

---

83 See *Cal. Evid. Code § 1160; Fla. Stat. Ann. § 90.4026; Tex. Civ. Prac. & Rem. Code § 18.061; Wash. Rev. Code § 5.66.010.*

84 *2003 Oregon Laws 384 (H.B. 3361 approved June 16, 2003).*

85 Id.

86 *2003 Colo. Legis. Serv. 126 (H.B. 03-1232 approved April 17, 2003).*

87 Id.

Note that this law applies to certain expressions regarding an "unanticipated outcome," which means "the outcome of a medical treatment or procedure that differs from an expected result."[88] The law applies to "health care providers," which include any person "licensed or certified by the state to deliver health care services" and a "clinic, health dispensary, or health facility licensed by the state of Colorado."[89]

So, the Colorado law applies to prevent the admission of the evidence described above (in bullet form) in "any civil action brought by an alleged victim of an unanticipated outcome of medical care, or in any arbitration proceeding related to such civil action."[90] However, one wonders whether such evidence would be admissible 1) in actions brought by a person other than the victim; 2) in actions brought by the alleged victim but not related to an "unanticipated outcome"—such as for fraud or an invasion of privacy or perhaps where the outcome was expected but the patient is otherwise unhappy; 3) in mediations (the state law only mentions arbitrations); or 4) in administrative proceedings—such as licensing board/licensure hearings.

The above two statutes provide some examples of successful legislative efforts. Other states may also be considering legislation that would encourage apologies by preventing the apologies from later being admitted as evidence against the apologizer.[91]

TIPS

1. Hospitals in states that have laws specifically protecting certain apologies or expressions of regret should consider including in their letters to patients, when appropriate, the words or phrases expressly protected by the state law, e.g., "regret."

2. A hospital also may wish to consider specifically labeling the top of the letter as being sent under the protective state law, e.g., "Sent Pursuant to Mass. Law § 23D."

88 Id.

89 Id.

90 Id.

91 See *Jonathan R. Cohen,* Legislating Apology: The Pros and Cons, *70 U. Cin. L. Rev. at 830.*

Offers To Compromise Or Settle A Dispute

Many states have laws that prevent an offer to compromise or settle a dispute from becoming an "admission" introduced as evidence against the maker of the offer.[92] Many of these states have identical (or very similar) language, excluding from evidence the 1) furnishing, offering, or promising to furnish, 2) the accepting, offering, or promising to accept, or 3) the attempting to compromise a claim that is disputed as to its amount or validity.[93] Some of these states also specifically protect attempts to resolve a claim through mediation or other alternative dispute resolution.[94] Note, however, that many of these state laws do permit a judge to admit this type of evidence "if offered for another purpose," such as proving a witness is biased or prejudiced, defending an allegation that one acted with undue delay, or proving an attempt to obstruct a criminal investigation or prosecution.[95]

Offering to pay another's hospital or medical expenses can be part of an effort to settle or compromise a dispute, and the evidence of such offer would generally not be introduced to a jury in a later lawsuit.[96] Additionally, the Federal Rules of Evidence (which apply in federal lawsuits) state evidence regarding the "furnishing or offering or promising to pay medical, hospital, or similar expenses occasioned by an injury is not admissible to prove liability for the injury."[97] This Federal Rule of Evidence also has exceptions and therefore does not always prevent such evidence from being admitted. Some of those exceptions include "when the evidence is offered for purposes other than proving liability or invalidity of the claim amount," as when proving bias or prejudice of

---

92 See *Ala. R. of Evid. 408; Alaska R. of Evid. 408; Ariz. R. of Evid. 408; Ark. Code Ann. § 16-41-101 (R. 408); Ark. R. of Evid. 408, Colo. R. of Evid. 408; Del. R. of Evid. 408; O.C.G.A. § 24-3-37 ("propositions made with a view to a compromise" are not admissions which can be admitted into evidence); Haw. R. of Evid. 408; Idaho R. of Evid. 408; Ind. R. of Evid. 408; Ky. R. of Evid. 408; La. R. of Evid. 408 (but not preventing such evidence to be admitted in criminal cases); Me. R. of Evid. 408; Md. R. of Evid. 5-408; Mich. R. of Evid. 408; Minn. R. of Evid. 408; Miss. R. of Evid. 408; Mont. R. of Evid. 408; Neb. R. of Evid. 27-408; N.H. R. of Evid. 408; N.J. R. of Evid. 408; N.M. R. of Evid. 11-408; N.C. R. of Evid. 408; N.D. R. of Evid. 408; Ohio R. of Evid. 408; Or. Rev. Stat. § 40.190 (R. 408); Pa. R. of Evid. 408; R.I. R. of Evid. 408; S.C. R. of Evid. 408; S.D. Codified Laws § 19-12-10 (R. 408); Tenn. R. of Evid. 408 (also stating "party may not be impeached by a prior inconsistent statement made in compromise negotiations"); Tex. R. of Evid. 408; Utah R. of Evid. 408; Vt. R. of Evid. 408; Wash. R. of Evid. 408; W.V. R. of Evid. 408; Wis. Stat. § 904.09; Wyoming R. of Evid. 408.*

93 Id.

94 See *Haw. R. of Evid. 408; Idaho R. of Evid. 408; Ind. R. of Evid. 408; Me. R. of Evid. 408; Md. R. of Evid. 5-408; Vt. R. of Evid. 408.*

95 See, e.g., Breedlove v. Aerotrim, U.S.A., Inc., *142 N.C. App. 447, 543 S.E.2d 213 (2001) (judge admitted portion of a tape-recorded conversation regarding negotiation of personal injury dispute for purpose of showing context of a later conversation).*

96 See, e.g., *735 Ill. Comp. Stat. 5/8-1901 (providing, paying or offering to pay for certain medical, hospital or other expenses is not an admission of liability; testimony, records, reports and other information or writings regarding such payment or offer is inadmissible, except when at the request of the person or persons who made such payment or offer).* See also Graziano v. Allen, *No. 02-2495, 2003 WL 21649499 (Wis. Ct. App. July 15, 2003) (in malpractice suit involving refractive eye surgeries, court properly excluded evidence the defendant eye surgeon offered to loan the patient money for the patient to obtain treatment from another physician).*

97 *Fed. R. Evid. 409.*

a witness, defending an allegation of undue delay, or showing an effort to obstruct a criminal investigation or prosecution—this list of exceptions is "not exclusive."[98]

Courts often exclude from evidence an offer to compromise a claim in an effort to encourage parties to resolve their disputes without litigation. In such cases, the defendant is trying to "settle" the matter, rather than trying to be benevolent, sympathetic or humanitarian. Note, however, such offers should not be for the full amount claimed by plaintiff; in other words, the offer should be a true compromise and should be for a claim which is disputed—disputed as to whether the claim is valid, what the amount of the claim is, or both.

For example, in a personal injury action, a court held an employer's letter admitting liability for a car accident should not be introduced into evidence because the letter "by its very terms, was written in an attempt to bring about mediation and compromise the claims in this case."[99] In another case, a court excluded from evidence the statement, "What is it going to take you make you folks happy?" on the basis such evidence was made "with a view to a compromise" by a company representative who was 1) attempting to resolve a dispute and 2) responsible for reviewing the investigation and assessing liability.[100] (It is obviously not the best practice to resolve patient complaints by asking, "What is it going to take to make you happy?") In another case, a hospital visitor slipped on the hospital stairs and fell on "remnants of a salad"; the hospital's associate administrator later wrote the visitor a letter in which he reviewed her allegations, summarized the results of the hospital's investigation and her condition, and offered to have an orthopedic specialist examine her and provide a treatment plan. The letter specifically offered to have the hospital "assume financial responsibility for your treatment should you avail yourself of our offer."[101] At trial, the judge excluded the letter from evidence, and the Court of Appeals approved because the letter constituted an offer of compromise.[102]

Also, a court might rule there must actually be a dispute in place before statements or admissions made while trying to compromise or settle such dispute will be protected from evidence. For example, offers to pay medical expenses of another person might not be protected as part of a compromise or settlement if the offer is made before a controversy or dispute actually arises.[103]

---

[98] See e.g.. Genova v. Longs Peak Emergency Physicians, P.C., *72 P.2d 454, 464 (Colo. Ct. App. 2003) (permitting letter to be admitted in order to rebut an allegation the plaintiff was entitled to punitive damages because the defendant had purportedly acted in a willful and wanton manner).*

[99] Mortensen v. Fowler-Flemister Concrete, Inc., *252 Ga. App. 395, 397-98, 555 S.E.2d 492, 494 (2001) (letter was sent by the defendant's lawyer to the plaintiff before trial; the letter admitted liability and that the only issue to address via mediation was damages; the case did not go to mediation but later proceeded to trial).*

[100] Houston v. Kinder-Care Learning Ctrs., Inc., *208 Ga. App. 235, 237, 430 S.E.2d 24, 26 (1993).*

[101] Burwell v. Easton Mem'l Hosp., *83 Md. App. 684, 691, 577 A.2d 394, 397 (1990).*

[102] Id.

[103] See Crain v. Allison, *443 A.2d 558, 565 (1982).*

For example, in one case, a court admitted evidence of a letter to a physician from the patient's husband and refused to find it was written as part of any settlement negotiations because "the parties were not engaged in a dispute at the time the letter was written ...."[104] Instead, for protection as a statement made with a view to compromise or settle, the parties should be attempting to settle an actual claim, controversy or dispute. Additionally, keep in mind the "settlement" should not be for the full amount of the claim, but for less than the full amount.[105]

Further, general or vague statements may not always be protected as made with a view to compromise or settle a dispute. As an example, after a drug overdose incident at a hospital, the hospital's CEO generally advised the patient's daughter to consult an attorney. At trial, the judge admitted evidence of the CEO's statements, and the Georgia Court of Appeals agreed, concluding the CEO's remarks were not made with a view to compromise because "no evidence showed that [the CEO] engaged in any efforts to compromise in these discussions."[106]

So, how can a hospital help show its communications with patients are made in of an effort to compromise or settle a dispute?

TIPS

1. Under the law of most states, hospitals can furnish, offer or promise to furnish money (or even a write off of a bill) as part of attempting to compromise or settle a disputed claim.
2. The amount offered should not be for the full amount of the claim; remember, the hospital is trying to reach a compromise.
3. Any correspondence communicating any such offer should be labeled "Privileged & Confidential—Offer to Compromise."
4. As extra protection, a hospital might consider labeling those portions of correspondence regarding a compromise with the citation (the reference number) for the law in that state protecting offers of compromise. Example: "Pursuant to Alabama Rule of Evidence 408."

---

104 Id. *at 566.*

105 Id. See also Stover v. Candle Corp. of Am., *238 Ga. App. 657, 658, 520 S.E.2d 7, 8 (1999) ("an unsolicited offer to settle for the full amount of the original claim is admissible").*

106 Hosp. Corp. of Lanier, Inc. v. Doster, *254 Ga. App. 169, 170, 561 S.E.2d 846, 849 (2002) (where a hospital admitted liability in giving a patient a drug overdose, the CEO's recommendation that the patient's family hire a lawyer was admissible because it was not part of settlement discussions.) The Georgia Court of Appeals also held evidence regarding the CEO's admissions of liability to the daughter was "harmless error" in a case, such as this one, where the hospital freely admitted to the jury it was liable for the drug overdose, concluding "[r]eferencing concessions of liability in settlement discussions cannot be harmful where the defendant concedes liability at trial." Id. at 171, 561 S.E.2d at 849.*

In many cases, contact between the hospital and the patient will take place over the phone, rather than through formal letters and bills. For example, the hospital may already have patient representatives who call patients to follow up after incidents or untoward complications occur. (In some hospitals, these representatives work in the Risk Management Department or may be patient advocates.) During these phone calls, patients can voice complaints and may request a write-off or reduction in their bill. If the hospital wishes to compromise (or settle) a matter by writing off a portion of the patient's bill, the hospital can take certain steps to show such action is not an admission of liability but is, instead, intended as an offer to compromise or settle the dispute.

TIPS

1. The hospital should consider labeling portions of bills showing write-offs or reductions as an "Offer to Compromise."
2. The hospital should label correspondence offering a write-off or reduction of bill in the same manner and consider citing to the state's law protecting such offers of compromise.

In other situations, it may be a hospital's practice to have a designated hospital representative contact a patient (or, if appropriate, a close family relative) to follow up regarding a complaint or incident at the hospital. Typically, someone at the hospital, such as the patient representative/advocate, might call the patient, say the hospital is performing routine follow up and ask how the patient is doing. The patient (or family relative) would then be given an opportunity to discuss the incident in full.

Figure 1.2

Tips for Phone Calls with Unhappy/ Complaining Patients

1. The hospital representative should document carefully the information given over the telephone to the patient, as well as the date and time of the phone call.
2. If the hospital representative is speaking with a person other than the patient, the representative should document the name of such person, their phone number and address, and the basis of their authority as an authorized representative of the patient.
3. The hospital representative should make sure he/she does not admit the hospital or others were negligent or liable; for example, the hospital may still be investigating the complaint. Consider using written guidelines (or even model scripts) of what should be discussed.
4. The hospital representative's goal in this call is to learn how the patient feels about the experience and possibly gauge whether the patient is still dissatisfied or might pursue a claim or lawsuit.
5. Therefore, the patient representative's job is to record information, rather than discuss the hospital's position regarding the complaint.
6. Because this type of contact with potentially unhappy patients requires finesse and consistency, hospitals should designate and train a few, specific personnel to telephone these patients.
7. During the call, the patient may express complaints or anger regarding the incident. The patient representative should be careful when making any apologies, but could say he/she apologizes for the patient's inconvenience.
8. If a patient voices a complaint that cannot be resolved, and if the patient has not already filed a complaint, the representative should consider reminding the patient of his or her right to submit a complaint to the hospital, the Medicare PRO and/or state survey agency.
9. The representative should write down the patient's comments and concerns (including any requests for write-offs of the bill) and could tell the patient the matter will be referred to "a committee" and someone will contact them again.

We know the patients' rights Condition of Participation requires the hospital's governing body (or a grievance committee) to "approve and be responsible for the effective operation of the grievance process" to "review and resolve grievances." A general example is set forth below as to how a patient representative could interact and work together effectively with a governing body or grievance committee (the reference to "committee" below includes a governing body or a grievance committee).[107]

[107] *For additional information regarding a process for receiving and reviewing patient complaints, see e.g., Patrice L. Spath,* Process for Handling Patient Grievances, *Brown-Spath & Associates, Sept. 2000, available at* www.brownspath.com/original_articles/grievances.htm.

Figure 1.3 General Tips Regarding Committee Involvement and Subsequent Follow Up with Patient Regarding Compromise

1. A hospital may wish to set a certain amount that the hospital can write off without involvement of a peer review committee. For example, if a case involves a nominal write-off or is otherwise below a certain amount (e.g., $250), the hospital could authorize a particular individual to approve the write-off.

2. If the state in which the hospital is located has a "peer review" statute, the governing body or grievance committee overseeing patient complaints should fit the definition of a "peer review committee" and may even be a peer review committee already established at the hospital. See, for example, O.C.G.A. § 31-7-131(1) (a Georgia law) (defining "peer review" to include medical audit, claims review,s and underwriting assistance).

3. At this peer review committee meeting (assuming state law recognizes the peer review privilege and the committee fits the state law criteria for a peer review committee), the members can discuss candidly whether the hospital has some liability, whether the hospital should pursue compromise and, if so, for how much. The committee may also wish to review information or documentation provided by the patient representative.

4. After the committee makes its decision, the hospital may wish to have the patient representative inform the patient of the decision via telephone and then follow up with sending the written notice required by the Hospital COP.

5. In that instance, the patient representative should document carefully this telephone call. The patient representative could tell the patient the hospital would like to reach a compromise and will reduce the bill by a certain amount, if the patient agrees. If the patient agrees, the hospital could then send the reduced bill labeled with the phrase "Offer to Compromise."

6. If the patient does not agree to a reduction or wants the bill reduced even more, then the matter could be referred back to the peer review committee. This committee could then determine whether the bill should be reduced even more or whether Risk Management and/or legal counsel should become involved.

7. If the amount of the proposed compromise or the incident/complaint is significant, a hospital should consider obtaining the patient's signature on a written release drafted by legal counsel, to ensure the write-off does not still allow the plaintiff to file suit against the hospital or others regarding the same incident.

It is impossible to predict whether a court will admit a hospital's offer of payment or compromise into evidence in a subsequent lawsuit. The clearer a defendant's liability, the greater the chance a court might find a defendant's offer of payment was an admission of liability. Therefore, in cases where the hospital has clear liability, the hospital should consider specifically describing its offers as views toward compromise that are not admissible into evidence. Note a hospital's offer might still be admissible to establish a separate issue at trial, such as the hospital's bad faith or stubborn litigiousness. Also, a hospital's offer may preclude or reduce the chance of obtaining summary judgment, since the offer may create an issue of fact. Nevertheless, the benefits of write-offs or compromises likely far outweigh the risks.

Cooperation clauses in health care providers' insurance policies

It's important to determine whether a hospital's actions in responding to a complaint—such as admitting responsibility in writing—could violate a "cooperation clause" in the hospital's liability insurance policy. Many insurance policies have "cooperation clauses" under which an insured agrees that it will cooperate with the insurance company regarding an incident or defense of a lawsuit. Other insurance policies are even more specific, requiring the insured not to admit liability or make any admissions; if such statements are made, the insurer may contend the insured violated the policy and assumed a financial obligation without the insurer's authorization. (Both types of clauses—those requiring cooperation and those prohibiting admissions—are referred to in this chapter together as "cooperation clauses.")

Cooperation clauses have been upheld and can require the cooperation of anyone who is "a defendant in a lawsuit or one who claims the benefit of insurance under the policy."[108] Basically, the purpose of a cooperation clause is to prevent collusion and to give the insurer complete control of the defense or compromise of suits or claims and to prevent, for example, willful acts which prevent an insurer from fully defending a claim or lawsuit, such as failing to show up for trial, failing to testify truthfully, not notifying the insurer, or settling claims without an insurer's approval.[109] Although these may be more "classic" examples of not cooperating with an insurance company, it is important to understand how courts have interpreted whether an admission of liability showed a lack of cooperation, such that the insurer was entitled to deny insurance coverage for the incident or the lawsuit.

In some cases, courts have held an insurance company was entitled to deny coverage (i.e., not pay) where an insured made certain admissions regarding liability or the other party's damages.[110] However, other courts have held an admission that merely recites factual events that occurred does not violate a policy's cooperation clause.[111]

---

[108] St. Paul Fire & Marine Ins. Co. v. Albany Emergency Ctr., *Inc., 184 Ga. App. 469, 470, 361 S.E.2d 687, 688 (1992).*

[109] See *44 Am. Jur. 2d Insurance § 1393 (2003).*

[110] See State Farm Mut. Ins. Co. v. Secrist, *33 P.3d 1272 (Colo. Ct. App. 2001) (finding insurer was entitled to deny coverage where the insured driver's admissions about the extent of the passenger's damages led to $100,000 judgment for which the insured driver, rather than the insurance company, would be responsible);* Youell v. Grimes, *217 F. Supp. 2d 1167 (D. Kan. 2002) (relieving insurer of contract liability where the insured breached a cooperation clause by admitting liability and increasing the settlement amount); and* Moore v. General Accident Ins. Co., *No. 92-1466, 1993 U.S. App. Lexis 5604 (4th Cir. Mar. 19, 1993) (confession of judgment violated a cooperation clause in an architect's professional liability policy).*

[111] See Monarch Ins. Co. v. Cook, *336 So. 2d 738 (Miss. 1976) (finding an insured's admission of liability related to sinking of a ship did not violate a cooperation clause, without proof of collusion between the claimant and the insured; also holding a cooperation clause does not require falsification of facts or putting up a sham defense);* Crook v. State Farm Mut. Auto Ins. Co., *235 S.C. 452, 112 S.E.2d 241 (1960) (holding a policy provision which prohibited an assumption of liability did not prohibit the insured party from giving the injured party a truthful explanation of the accident. Note, however, that the court found the insurer suffered no prejudice by a truthful explanation, because it insured both parties).*

In other cases, an insurance company must show the insured's lack of cooperation actually prejudiced the insurer's ability to defend its case.[112] However, in some states, courts have held an insurer is not required to show it was prejudiced by an insured's willful and unjustified violation of a policy's cooperation clause.[113] Additionally, states may have different laws, including court decisions, which may address cooperation clauses and what an insurance company must prove in order to show a lack of cooperation sufficient to deny coverage.

TIPS

1. A hospital should review all of its insurance policies (including excess insurance) and identify whether the policies contain a cooperation or anti-admissions clause.
2. Before an incident occurs, a hospital should talk with its insurance company now about such clauses in the hospital's policies. Discuss the clauses and the insurance company's position and identify mutually agreeable options. (As a starting point for discussions, for example, the hospital could mention to the insurance company the JCAHO standard for disclosing unanticipated outcomes.)
3. Before admitting liability to a patient or family for a particular incident, a hospital should strongly consider talking with its insurance company first.
4. A hospital should also be aware of its state's laws regarding these cooperation clauses and consult an insurance lawyer as needed.

---

[112] See e.g., Union Ins. Co. v. Williams, *261 F. Supp. 2d 1150 (E.D. Mo. 2003).*

[113] See e.g., KHD Deutz of Am. Corp. v. UTICA Mut. Ins. Co., *220 Ga. App. 194, 469 S.E.2d 336 (1996).*

CHAPTER 2

HIPAA and Patient Complaints: What to Consider

CHAPTER 2

HIPAA and Patient Complaints: What to Consider

Background

The Health Insurance Portability and Accountability Act of 1996 (HIPAA) provides widespread health care regulation addressing the privacy and security of patient protected health information. In addition, HIPAA allows patients certain rights with regard to their protected health information (PHI). One of these is the right to file a privacy-related complaint with both the health care organization and the secretary of the Department of Health and Human Services (HHS). Health care organizations must ensure that they have established a privacy complaint policy and process as well as provided education to workforce members on responding appropriately to privacy-related complaints. It is in the best interest of the health care organization to respond in a timely and appropriate manner to the complainant of a privacy-related complaint to avoid later involvement with HHS or other external accrediting or licensure agencies.

Chapter objectives:

- Provide a framework for developing guidelines for managing privacy-related complaints
- Identify necessary steps for investigating and resolving privacy-related complaints
- Recognize internal resources for investigating and resolving privacy-related complaints
- Distinguish the involvement of external agencies that may be involved in resolving privacy-related complaints
- Develop a template for written responses to privacy-related complaints

Developing guidelines and policies for managing privacy-related complaints

Each organization must have in place a process for responding to patient privacy complaints. Ideally an organizational policy has been developed to provide guidance to staff receiving and responding to privacy complaints. Once the policy has been developed, appropriate staff education is required to ensure that each privacy complaint is responded to in a manner that best meets the needs of the individual bringing forth the complaint. The policy should include the following elements identified in bold text:

1. **Title**: Choose a title that reflects guidance for privacy-related complaints
2. **Policy Statement**: Explain [Organization Name]'s policy for responding to all complaints raised with regard to privacy-related issues brought forth by patients, visitors, staff, or other internal/external sources
3. **Purpose**: Reason why the policy has been created
4. **Background**: Reference to internal and external influences that impact the policy (HIPAA)
5. **See Also**: List other supporting documents and policies
6. **Attachments**: List supporting attachments/forms including investigative record, sample log entry
7. **Definitions**: Define all pertinent definitions including PHI
8. **Procedures**: List all steps
9. **Approval**: Names, titles, and dates
10. **Distribution List**: List relevant departments affected
11. **Review Dates**: List as appropriate
12. **Sources**: List all references used for policy development
13. **Applicable Standards and Regulations**: List pertinent federal and state regulations (HIPAA)

Once the policy has been developed, the health care organization must provide training and education to workforce members on the policy and process for addressing privacy related complaints. Workforce members must be aware of the appropriate response to a patient's privacy complaint as well as the internal process for referring the complaint to the appropriate person/department for investigation and resolution.

Identifying necessary steps for investigating and resolving privacy-related complaints

The organization may already have in place a process for handling patient complaints and this may be expanded to encompass privacy complaints. The organization may also choose to handle these complaints separately. Regardless of the process for handling the complaints, a log should be established to record all privacy-related complaints. Information collected for the log should be basic and brief in description. A sample log entry should include:

- Datc of complaint
- Source of complaint/name of complainant
- Brief description of complaint (details to be saved for investigative record)
- Name of individual receiving complaint
- Resolution of complaint—brief statement
- Follow-up—if applicable

Figure 2.1 Sample Privacy-Related Complaints Log Entry

COMPLAINT INFORMATION		Complaint #:	Org.:
Date of Complaint			
Source of Complaint			
Description Of Complaint			
Received By/ Investigated By			
Resolution:			
Follow-Up:			

A complaint investigation record should include the detailed information regarding the receipt, investigation, resolution, and follow-up of the complaint. Any additional documentation/correspondence should be maintained with the investigation record. Figure 2.2 provides a sample.

Figure 2.2 **Sample Privacy-Related Complaints Investigation Record**

Complainant's Name ______________________ **Log #:** __________

Telephone #: ______________ **Date of Report:** ______________

Taken By: ______________ **Investigated By:** ______________

Summary of Complaint

____

____

____

____

Summary of Investigation & Follow-Up

____

____

____

____

Resolution Steps:

- ❑ Documented in privacy complaint log
- ❑ Follow-up provided in writing to complainant within 30 days (if not, document reason)
- ❑ Notification made to other concerned parties including:
  - Legal/RM issue: local administration, risk management coordinator, integrity officer
  - DHHS complaint: local administration, risk management coordinator, integrity officer; corporate VP of mission & culture integration, corporate director of privacy, corporate director of reimbursement & compliance
- ❑ Original complaint and all investigation documentation attached

Completed By: ______________________ **Date:** ______________

Figure 2.3 **Top 10 Tips for Managing Privacy-Related Complaints**

The following steps are key in managing a privacy-related complaint and should be incorporated into the organizational policy and procedures under the investigation process/procedures:

1. Respond in a timely manner
2. Respond with a professional, compassionate, and courteous manner
3. Listen actively—do not interrupt or get defensive
4. Show empathy and understanding; acknowledge the complainant's feelings
5. Ask questions to clarify the issue
6. Determine what the complainant wants
7. Discuss alternative solutions/options
8. Take action
9. Keep complainant informed of progress/provide feedback on resolution in writing
10. Follow-up to ensure satisfaction

Note: Document on the report form the information you gather (related to the above) as part of the investigation process.

Recognizing internal resources for investigating and resolving privacy-related complaints

Organizations may have in place established programs and policy/procedures for responding to patient complaints and may incorporate privacy-related complaints into the already existing processes. Other organizations may choose to have these privacy complaints managed by the privacy officer. Regardless of how the privacy complaints are managed, it is critical that the privacy officer has a lead role in the investigation and response to the complaint. Other key resources within the organization may provide assistance and guidance in investigating and resolving privacy complaints and should be kept aware of privacy issues that may impact the organization. These resources may include staff from the following departments:

- Senior leadership members (administration, board of directors, medical staff president)
- Human resources department director
- Legal counsel
- Risk management coordinator
- Compliance officer
- Public relations/media relations coordinator

Distinguishing the involvement of external agencies in resolving privacy-related complaints

The timely response and investigation of a privacy complaint on the part of a health care organization may contain the complaint to the local level and prevent involvement of external governmental, licensing, and/or accrediting agencies. The Privacy Rule clearly defines the patient right to file a privacy complaint not only with the health care organization, but also with HHS. Complaints filed with HHS will be turned over to the Office for Civil Rights (OCR) for investigation and resolution. Any individual, who believes that a health care organization is not complying with the privacy rule, may file a complaint with the Secretary of HHS. The complaint must be submitted in writing, must name the health care organization that is the subject of the complaint, and describe acts or omissions believed to be in violation. The complaint must be filed within 180 days of when the complainant know or should have known that the act or omission occurred. Investigation may include a review of the pertinent policies, procedures, or practices of the covered entity and of the circumstances regarding any alleged acts or omissions concerning compliance. Should it be determined that the complaint is valid, financial penalties may be imposed upon the health care organization.

Additionally, a patient may also file a privacy related complaint with the Joint Commission on Accreditation of Healthcare Organizations (JCAHO). JCAHO may choose to investigate the complaint through an unannounced on-site survey. Should the JCAHO validate the complaint, it may impose recommendations for improvements upon the health care organization.

Lastly, a patient may also involve their state licensing bureau or any other state office responsible for the oversight of health care organizations. Like JCAHO, the state may choose to investigate the complaint through an unannounced on-site survey and may impose fines and sanctions.

Facts about how patients can file a privacy complaint with the OCR

Your hospital or state may require you to share information with patients about how they can report a privacy violation. Therefore we've included information about how to do this as well as a copy of the actual Health Information Privacy Complaint form. Some hospitals do include this form with correspondence to complainants in cases of privacy-related complaints.

Anyone can file written complaints with OCR by mail, fax, or e-mail. If you have a question about the complaint form, you may call the OCR toll free number: 1-800-368-1019. OCR has ten regional offices, and each regional office covers certain states. Complaints should be sent to the appropriate OCR Regional Office, based on the region where the alleged violation took place. You may find the OCR office list at this Web site: *www.hhs.gov/ocr/privacyhowtofile.htm*

Complainants should ensure that their written complaint contains the following information[1]:

- Name, full address, home and work telephone numbers, e-mail address.
- If you are filing a complaint on someone's behalf, also provide the name of the person on whose behalf you are filing.
- Name, full address and telephone number of the person, agency or organization you believe violated your (or someone else's) health information privacy rights or committed another violation of the Privacy Rule.
- Briefly describe what happened. How, why, and when do you believe your (or someone else's) health information privacy rights were violated, or the Privacy Rule otherwise was violated?
- Any other relevant information.
- Please sign your name and date your letter.
- The following information is optional:
  - Do you need special accommodations for us to communicate with you about this complaint?
  - If we cannot reach you directly, is there someone else we can contact to help us reach you?
  - Have you filed your complaint somewhere else?

---

[1] *Material quoted from: OCR Fact Sheet: How To File A Health Information Privacy Complaint With The Office For Civil Rights,* www.hhs.gov/ocr/privacyhowtofile.htm

Complainants have three options for submitting complaints to the OCR [2]:

If you mail or fax the complaint, be sure to follow the instructions above for determining the correct regional office.

Option 1: Open and print out the *Health Information Privacy Complaint Form* in PDF format (you will need Adobe Acrobat Reader software) at *www.hhs.gov/ocr/howtofileprivacy.pdf* and fill it out. Return the completed complaint to the appropriate OCR Regional Office by mail or fax.

Option 2: Download the *Health Information Privacy Complaint Form* in Microsoft Word format to your own computer from *www.hhs.gov/ocr/howtofileprivacy.doc*, fill out and save the form using Microsoft Word. Use the Tab and Shift/Tab on your keyboard to move from field to field in the form. Then, you can either: (a) print the completed form and mail or fax it to the appropriate OCR Regional Office; or (b) e-mail the form to OCR at OCR*Complaint@hhs.gov.*

Option 3: If you choose not to use the OCR-provided *Health Information Privacy Complaint Form* (although we recommend that you do), please provide the information specified above and either: (a) send a letter or fax to the appropriate OCR Regional Office; or (b) send an email to OCR at OCR*Complaint@hhs.gov.*

If you require an answer regarding a general health information privacy question, please view our Frequently Asked Questions (FAQs). If you still need assistance, you may call OCR (toll-free) at: 1-866-627-7748. You may also send an email to OCR*Privacy@hhs.gov* with suggestions regarding future FAQs. E-mails will not receive individual responses.

---

[2] *Material quoted from: OCR Fact Sheet: How To File A Health Information Privacy Complaint With The Office For Civil Rights,* www.hhs.gov/ocr/privacyhowtofile.htm

Figure 2.4 **OCR Health Information Privacy Complaint**

Form Approved: OMB No. 0990-0269
See OMB Statement on Reverse.

DEPARTMENT OF HEALTH AND HUMAN SERVICES
OFFICE FOR CIVIL RIGHTS (OCR)
HEALTH INFORMATION PRIVACY COMPLAINT

If you have questions about this form, call OCR (toll-free) at:
1-800-368-1019 (any language) or 1-800-537-7697 (TDD)

YOUR FIRST NAME		YOUR LAST NAME
HOME PHONE ( )		WORK PHONE ( )
STREET ADDRESS		CITY
STATE	ZIP	E-MAIL ADDRESS *(If available)*

Are you filing this complaint for someone else? ☐ Yes ☐ No

If Yes, whose health information privacy rights do you believe were violated?

FIRST NAME	LAST NAME

Who (or what agency or organization, e.g., provider, health plan) do you believe violated your (or someone else's) health information privacy rights or committed another violation of the Privacy Rule?

PERSON/AGENCY/ORGANIZATION

STREET ADDRESS		CITY
STATE	ZIP	PHONE ( )

When do you believe that the violation of health information privacy rights occurred?

LIST DATE(S)

Describe briefly what happened. How and why do you believe your (or someone else's) health information privacy rights were violated, or the privacy rule otherwise was violated? Please be as specific as possible. *(Attach additional pages as needed)*

Please sign and date this complaint.

SIGNATURE	DATE

Filing a complaint with OCR is voluntary. However, without the information requested above, OCR may be unable to proceed with your complaint. We collect this information under authority of the Privacy Rule issued pursuant to the Health Insurance Portability and Accountability Act of 1996. We will use the information you provide to determine if we have jurisdiction and, if so, how we will process your complaint. Information submitted on this form is treated confidentially and is protected under the provisions of the Privacy Act of 1974. Names or other identifying information about individuals are disclosed when it is necessary for investigation of possible health information privacy violations, for internal systems operations, or for routine uses, which include disclosure of information outside the Department for purposes associated with health information privacy compliance and as permitted by law. It is illegal for a covered entity to intimidate, threaten, coerce, discriminate or retaliate against you for filing this complaint or for taking any other action to enforce your rights under the Privacy Rule. You are not required to use this form. You also may write a letter or submit a complaint electronically with the same information. To submit an electronic complaint, go to our web site at: **www.hhs.gov/ocr/privacyhowtofile.html**. To mail a complaint see reverse page for OCR Regional addresses.

HHS-700 (4/03) (FRONT)

Figure 2.4 OCR Health Information Privacy Complaint (cont.)

(The remaining information on this form is optional. Failure to answer these voluntary questions will not affect OCR's decision to process your complaint.)

Do you need special accommodations for us to communicate with you about this complaint (check all that apply)?

☐ Braille ☐ Large Print ☐ Cassette tape ☐ Computer diskette ☐ Electronic mail ☐ TDD

☐ Sign language interpreter *(specify language)*: ______________________

☐ Foreign language interpreter *(specify language)*: ______________________ ☐ Other: ______________

If we cannot reach you directly, is there someone we can contact to help us reach you?

FIRST NAME	LAST NAME
HOME PHONE ( )	WORK PHONE ( )
STREET ADDRESS	CITY
STATE / ZIP	E-MAIL ADDRESS *(If available)*

Have you filed your complaint anywhere else? If so, please provide the following. (Attach additional pages as needed.)

PERSON / AGENCY / ORGANIZATION / COURT NAME(S)

DATE(S) FILED	CASE NUMBER(S) *(If known)*

To help us better serve the public, please provide the following information for the person you believe had their health information privacy rights violated (you or the person on whose behalf you are filing).

ETHNICITY *(select one)*

☐ Hispanic or Latino

☐ Not Hispanic or Latino

RACE *(select one or more)*

☐ American Indian or Alaska Native ☐ Asian ☐ Native Hawaiian or Other Pacific Islander

☐ Black or African American ☐ White ☐ Other *(specify)*: ______________

PRIMARY LANGUAGE SPOKEN *(if other then English)*	HOW DID YOU LEARN ABOUT THE OFFICE FOR CIVIL RIGHTS?

To mail a complaint, please type or print, and return completed complaint to the OCR Regional Address based on the region where the alleged discrimination took place.

Region I - CT, ME, MA, NH, RI, VT Office for Civil Rights Department of Health & Human Services JFK Federal Building - Room 1875 Boston, MA 02203 (617) 565-1340; (617) 565-1343 (TDD) (617) 565-3809 FAX	**Region V - IL, IN, MI, MN, OH, WI** Office for Civil Rights Department of Health & Human Services 233 N. Michigan Ave. - Suite 240 Chicago, IL 60601 (312) 886-2359; (312) 353-5693 (TDD) (312) 886-1807 FAX	**Region IX - AZ, CA, HI, NV, AS, GU, The U.S. Affiliated Pacific Island Jurisdictions** Office for Civil Rights Department of Health & Human Services 50 United Nations Plaza - Room 322 San Francisco, CA 94102 (415) 437-8310; (415) 437-8311 (TDD) (415) 437-8329 FAX
Region II - NJ, NY, PR, VI Office for Civil Rights Department of Health & Human Services 26 Federal Plaza - Suite 3313 New York, NY 10278 (212) 264-3313; (212) 264-2355 (TDD) (212) 264-3039 FAX	**Region VI - AR, LA, NM, OK, TX** Office for Civil Rights Department of Health & Human Services 1301 Young Street - Suite 1169 Dallas, TX 75202 (214) 767-4056; (214) 767-8940 (TDD) (214) 767-0432 FAX	
Region III - DE, DC, MD, PA, VA, WV Office for Civil Rights Department of Health & Human Services 150 S. Independence Mall West - Suite 372 Philadelphia, PA 19106-3499 (215) 861-4441; (215) 861-4440 (TDD) (215) 861-4431 FAX	**Region VII - IA, KS, MO, NE** Office for Civil Rights Department of Health & Human Services 601 East 12th Street - Room 248 Kansas City, MO 64106 (816) 426-7278; (816) 426-7065 (TDD) (816) 426-3686 FAX	**Region X - AK, ID, OR, WA** Office for Civil Rights Department of Health & Human Services 2201 Sixth Avenue - Mail Stop RX-11 Seattle, WA 98121 (206) 615-2290; (206) 615-2296 (TDD) (206) 615-2297 FAX
Region IV - AL, FL, GA, KY, MS, NC, SC, TN Office for Civil Rights Department of Health & Human Services 61 Forsyth Street, SW. - Suite 3B70 Atlanta, GA 30323 (404) 562-7886; (404) 331-2867 (TDD) (404) 562-7881 FAX	**Region VIII - CO, MT, ND, SD, UT, WY** Office for Civil Rights Department of Health & Human Services 1961 Stout Street - Room 1426 Denver, CO 80294 (303) 844-2024; (303) 844-3439 (TDD) (303) 844-2025 FAX	

Burden Statement

Public reporting burden for the collection of information on this complaint form is estimated to average 45 minutes per response, including the time for reviewing instructions, gathering the data needed and entering and reviewing the information on the completed complaint form. An agency may not conduct or sponsor, and a person is not required to respond to, a collection of information unless it displays a valid control number. Send comments regarding this burden estimate or any other aspect of this collection of information, including suggestions for reducing this burden, to: HHS/OS Reports Clearance Officer, Office of Information Resources Management, 200 Independence Ave. S.W., Room 531H, Washington, D.C. 20201.

HHS-700 (4/03) (BACK)

Developing a template for written responses to privacy related complaints

If the investigation of the complaint is carried out in a thorough and timely manner, then developing a written response to the complainant should follow easily. The written response should:

- Thank the complainant for bringing the privacy concern to the attention of the health care organization.
- Indicate the organization's commitment to responding to the concern.
- Recap the complainant's concern as it was recorded by the organization.
- Identify the actions that the organization took to investigate and the corrective actions to resolve the concern and prevent future occurrences. This should be done using broad and non-specific language such as "process-improvement," "employee counseling," "revision of existing policies and procedures," etc.
- Once again, thank the complainant for the opportunity to improve the organization's operations.
- Offer additional support and contact information for future services.

Figure 2.5 Sample Privacy Complaint/Concern Letter: Privacy Issue

[Insert Date]

[Insert Patient/Representative's Address]

Dear [Insert Patient/Representative's Name]:

Thank you for contacting [Insert Organization's Name] and sharing with us your concern regarding our patient privacy practices. We are committed to protecting the privacy of the patient health information we collect and continuously work toward improving our processes and systems to ensure that this information is safeguarded.

Based on your communications with [Insert Organization's Name] focused on the following information [recap the individual's privacy concern].

To address this issue, we investigated [provide a brief explanation of the process in broad generic statements].

As a result, we have [provide information regarding corrective action processes, procedural change, employee education and/or counseling, etc., in broad generic statements].

At [Insert Organization's Name], we continuously strive to provide high quality patient care in a confidential and secure manner. It is our hope that this letter communicates to you our continued commitment in meeting your needs and continuously improving our services.

If I can be of any additional assistance, please do not hesitate to contact me [Insert Phone Number]. Again, thank you for taking the time to communicate your concerns to us. We will use your feedback anonymously and constructively to improve our privacy practices.

Sincerely,

[Insert Local Privacy Officer/Respondent's Name]

Figure 2.6

Sample Privacy Complaint/Concern Letter: Notice of Privacy Practices

[Insert Date]

[Insert Patient/Representative's Address]

Dear [Insert Patient/Representative's Name]:

Thank you for your inquiry regarding the [Insert Organization's Name] Notice of Privacy Practices. As required by the Health Insurance Portability and Accountability Act of 1996 (HIPAA), [Insert Organization's Name] has published within the Notice of Privacy Practices an overview of our privacy practices as well as our patients' privacy rights.

Federal regulations (HIPAA) were recently passed to provide greater protections for patient privacy as well as requiring health care providers to identify uses and disclosures of patient health information. We are committed to protecting patient privacy and working well within the regulations provided at both the federal and state level.

Your concerns centered on the following issues. I will do my best to respond to these concerns and provide additional supporting information.

[Begin customization here to address specific concern(s). Select one or more of the following paragraphs as appropriate to address patient/representative concern(s) to include in your letter.]

Use of Patient Information for Organ Donation Purposes
Health care providers at [Insert Organization's Name] are required by law to work with organ donation activities upon the death of a patient when the patient has either previously indicated his/her status as an organ donor or the patient's personal representative has consented to organ donation. Information would not be released unless the above conditions existed. While this is requirement is part of the federal "Conditions of Participation" for health care providers, it is also covered in [Insert State Name], Statute – [Insert Reference].

Use of Patient Information for Research Purposes
[Insert Organization's Name] will only use your patient-specific information for internal research purposes with your prior authorization. Health care providers are required by law to have in

Figure 2.6

Sample Privacy Complaint/Concern Letter: Notice of Privacy Practices (cont.)

place policies and practices that address the use of patient information for research activities. [Insert Organization's Name] will not share patient information for external research projects without patient authorization.

Use of Patient Information for Marketing Purposes
HIPAA defines "marketing" as making a communication about a product or service that encourages recipient of the communication to purchase or use the product or service, unless the communication is made to describe a health-related product or service that is provided by the health care organization making the communication. Patients who may have previously agreed to the receipt of marketing materials under these circumstances have the ability to "opt-out" and request that [Insert Organization's Name] no longer forward to them marketing information as defined above. [Insert Organization's Name] will not share or sell patient name listings to other agencies for purposes of marketing.

[Insert Organization's Name] will continue to use mass mailings to communicate our products and services. These materials are not considered "marketing" under HIPAA and we will continue our practices of providing newsletters and announcements to our patients and the public. Examples of communications that are not considered "marketing" and to not require [Insert Organization's Name] to provide an "opt-out" option are communications to promote health in a general manner and do not promote a specific product or service. Examples may include communications

- reminding women to get an annual mammogram
- about health education or disease prevention
- regarding support groups, cancer prevention, and health fairs
- in informative newsletter formats

Many communications of this type are based on external community-based mailing lists and not patient listings.

Use of Patient Information for Fundraising Purposes
HIPAA allows health care organizations to use very basic patient information without patient authorization for fundraising activities carried out for the organization. The only patient information used or disclosed is: name, address, age, gender, insurance status, and/or dates of

Figure 2.6

Sample Privacy Complaint/Concern Letter: Notice of Privacy Practices (cont.)

service. Patient authorization is required for any fundraising activities that involve information beyond what is identified above. Written communications sent out for purposes of fundraising must also include information as to how to allow the recipient to "opt-out" of receiving any future fundraising communications, regardless of whether the recipients name was acquired through the organization's patient database or acquired through a public database.

At your request, [Insert Organization's Name] will be happy to remove your name from communications that involve fundraising activities.

[Optional statement for your organization:]

At the present time, [Insert Organization's Name] is not actively using patient information for any fundraising activities.

Patients' Right to Request Restrictions on How Protected Health Information is Used and Disclosed
As noted in the Notice of Privacy Practices, our patients have the right to request restrictions on how protected health information is used and disclosed. We will be happy to review a request for restrictions and determine appropriate action.

[End customization here after addressing patient/representative concern(s).]

We appreciate your questions and concerns regarding our Notice of Privacy Practices and how we protect, use and disclosure your health information. As we move forward with our HIPAA compliance efforts, we will continue to improve how we communicate our practices. The Notice is truly an overview and required by law. We did our best to try and condense the hundreds of pages of privacy policies, procedures, and practices into a concise document.

At [Insert Organization's Name], we continuously strive to provide high quality patient care in a confidential and secure manner. We have invested in privacy training for all staff members. Additionally we have worked to develop comprehensive privacy policies that ensure protection of health information.

Figure 2.6

Sample Privacy Complaint/Concern Letter: Notice of Privacy Practices (cont.)

It is our hope that this letter further clarifies our position. Unfortunately, it is very difficult to address all privacy practices in the Notice. Our goal was to develop a notice that provided a broad overview and was patient friendly. We recognize that we will need to continue to refine the Notice as patients provide us with helpful comments and feedback.

If I can be of any additional assistance, please do not hesitate to contact me [Insert Phone Number]. Again, thank you for taking the time to communicate your concerns to us. We will use your feedback anonymously and constructively to improve our privacy practices.

Sincerely,

[Insert Local Privacy Officer/Respondent's Name]

CHAPTER 3

Policies, Procedures and Forms: Samples

CHAPTER 3

Policies, Procedures and Forms: Samples

This chapter contains examples of policies, procedures, and forms for responding to patient dissatisfaction.

Figure 3.1

Heritage Valley Health System Administrative Policies and Procedures

Subject: Process for Handling Customer Complaints **Policy Number:** Adm.1.27

Uniquely connected. For life.℠ HERITAGE VALLEY Health System

Sponsor: Organizational Performance Team **Effective Date:** July 2001
Revised Date: January 2003

Policy

It is the policy of the hospitals of Heritage Valley Health System (HVHS) to deliver quality medical care to all patients. It is the policy of the hospitals of HVHS to provide a process for handling complaints when the patient, family member, or visitor is less than satisfied with services rendered. This procedure will provide a process whereby complaints can be registered. Every complaint will be distributed to the appropriate management staff. Investigation and problem resolution will follow and the customer will be contacted in a timely fashion with the results of the complaint process. Should the customer be dissatisfied with the results of this process, a method for grievance is provided which will include the Chief Operating Officer and the Vice President/Chief Medical Officer. Protected Health Information (PHI) is managed per state and federal regulations, including but not limited to, the Health Insurance Portability and Accountability Act of 1996 (HIPAA).

Instructions

Responsibility	*Action*
Patient, Family Member, or Visitor	1. Contacts HVHS verbally, via mail, or electronically to register a complaint.
HVHS Personnel	2. Receives complaint. 3. Informs customer the complaint will be investigated and followed up in a timely manner. 4. Forwards complaint to the appropriate management personnel as determined by referencing contact list in Public Folders under Department Shared Information. If in-person communication with manager is not possible, dial organizational performance team (OPT) support services at [insert telephone number].

Figure 3.1

Heritage Valley Health System Administrative Policies and Procedures (cont.)

(If contacted) OPT	5. Addresses complaint with customer, collecting pertinent information. 6. Forwards complaint information to manager.
Management Personnel	7. Receives complaint. 8. Documents complaint on Customer Comment Form. (Located in Public Folder—Department Shared Information.) 9. Conducts investigation of complaint. 10. Corrects identified problems where possible. 11. Provides written follow up to customer within two weeks of initiation of complaint, when identification provided. (Response Letter Template is available in Public Folders—Department-Shared Information folder.) 12. Forwards results of investigation and follow up to Vice President and OPT
OPT - Organizational Performance Team	13. Informs the Vice President about customers who are not satisfied with resolution or explanation.
Vice President	14. Contacts customer and attempts to resolve. 15. If customer remains dissatisfied, informs customer of grievance process. 16. Forwards updated customer comment form to Chief Operating Officer.
Chief Operating Officer	17. Reviews issue with appropriate administrative staff and attempts resolution with patient or family. 18. If not successful, convenes Grievance Committee including appropriate staff; (i.e., Chief Medical Officer, Operational Managers, Risk Management, etc.).
Grievance Committee	19. Reviews grievance issue. 20. Determines appropriate action and renders decision on grievance within two weeks of receipt. 21. Informs customer of grievance outcome in writing. 22. Submits copy of outcome to Organizational Performance Team.
OPT	23. Ensures investigation and follow up are complete. 24. Trends results of complaint process. 25. Files complaint and outcome.

Figure 3.2

Heritage Valley Health System
Sample Customer Comment Form

CUSTOMER COMMENT FORM

Date:

To: (Name of manager)

cc: (Vice President)
OPT Support Services Log

Re: (Enter the word–Compliment or Complaint)

Patient Name		Room # (if applicable)	
Respondent (if other than Patient)		Discharge or Date of Service	
Address		Telephone #	
Response Required		Survey # (if applicable)	

Complaint: Activate Problem Solving Process, attempt to complete within two weeks of notification. Document Problem Solving measures, and follow-up. File in Department's Customer Comment file and forward copy of report to Manager, Vice Pres. & Dir. OPT Support Services.

Comments:

Documentation of Action Taken:

Date Closing Letter sent:
Date Completed:
Name of Staff Completing Form:

Figure 3.3

Sample Patient Complaint Process from Eastern State Hospital

EASTERN STATE HOSPITAL
Williamsburg, Virginia

QUALITY MANAGEMENT
[Number]
[Date]

SUBJECT: Patient Complaint Process

REFERENCE:

1. DMHMRSAS, rules and regulations to ensure the rights of individuals receiving services from providers of mental health, mental retardation and substance abuse services.
2. Eastern State Hospital policy statement, patient's rights and access to the patient advocate, [number]
3. Eastern State Hospital policy statement, reporting and investigating abuse and neglect of clients, [number]

RESPONSIBILITY: **All Eastern State Hospital staff**

POLICY:

Every attempt will be made to resolve a patient's rights complaint to the individual's satisfaction at the earliest possible step. No action will be taken, permitted, or condoned to retaliate against or prevent anyone from filing a complaint or helping a patient to file a complaint. Staff will assist the complainant in understanding the full complaint process, the options for the resolution, and the elements of confidentiality. The individual or legally authorized representatives may contact the advocate at anytime to pursue a formal complaint. In the complaint process, anyone who knows of or has reason to believe that a patient may have been abused, neglected, or exploited at any location shall immediately report directly to the hospital director.

Procedure:

1. Patient complaints (expression of dissatisfaction, grievance or concern) communicated to their treatment team or any hospital staff, that can be resolved in the building or by the treatment team or hospital staff will be resolved at that level.

2. If the complaint cannot be resolved the patient has a right to submit a complaint using attachment (A) directly to the patient complaint liaison (PCL). The patient also can call the PCL with the complaint.

NUMBER: [number]

3. If so requested, ESH staff will assist the patient in filling out the attached patient complaint form(s) to be forwarded or faxed to the PCL in [office detail]. If the patient does not desire to fill out the form, the option of calling the PCL will be made available to the patient. On behalf of the hospital director, the PCL will investigate the complaint with the authority from the director to negotiate resolutions when appro-

Figure 3.3

Sample Patient Complaint Process from Eastern State Hospital (cont.)

priate with the department heads. If the complaint involves patient safety or facility safety issues and the patient is in danger of injury, immediate action will be taken to correct the situation.

4. The PCL will meet with the patient the next working day after the complaint is received day regarding his/her complaint to clarify any issues and to inform the patient that his/her complaint has been received and will be addressed.

5. The complaint will be entered into the automated patient complaint program with the proposed resolution. The PCL will then meet with the patient and provide him with a copy of attachment (B) with the resolution. He will also discuss with the patient the resolution in detail. The patient may sign the patient complaint form(s) and indicate whether he is satisfied with the resolution. The PCL will document the patient's response to the resolution on the complaint form and enter the response in the automated patient complaint program. The PCL will keep a copy.

6. Not all complaints will necessarily require a solution. However, all complaints will be reviewed.

7. The hospital has five (5) working days after receipt of a complaint to address the issue and present a resolution to the patient.

8. If the patient and or legally authorized representative, as applicable, is not satisfied with the resolution, then the director or PCL shall immediately notify the human rights advocate.

9. Complaints that are not resolved in five (5) working days will become a formal complaint and forwarded to the human rights advocate for substantial risk review.

10. If found to be of substantial risk the human rights advocate will inform the hospital director who will follow ESH policy for abuse and DI-201 or take other action as deemed appropriate. The human rights advocate will inform the LHRC and the LHRC shall conduct a hearing according to the special procedure as out-lined in 12VAC 35-115-170.

NUMBER: [number]

11. If NOT found to be of substantial risk the human rights advocate will return the complaint to the PCL who will attempt to resolve the complaint by meeting with the patient within 24 hours.

Figure 3.3

Sample Patient Complaint Process from Eastern State Hospital (cont.)

12. If unable to resolve the complaint an investigation will be done with an action plan forwarded to the patient within 10 working days.

13. The patient has five (5) working days to respond verbally and/or in writing to the action plan suggested.

14. The director has 10 days to respond to the patient and human rights advocate concerning the final resolution.

15. If the patient is not satisfied, the patient with the involvement of the human rights advocate may petition the LHRC for a hearing on a decision concerning the complaint.

16. The PCL will report monthly any trends identified to the director of quality management, the hospital director and the human rights advocate.

    These reports will include any identified trends along with recommendations as appropriate. The director of quality management, the hospital director and the human rights advocate will have access to the automated patient complaint program to review all patient complaints, the proposed resolution and data trends for each patient care building and category of complaint.

17. The PCL will do a 30-day follow-up to ensure the resolutions are in place.

18. Patient complaint posters will be posted in all patient care areas. Attachment (C).

Hospital Director ____________________

DRR
6/12/02
Attachments: A: Patient Complaint Form
B. Computer Generated Patient Complaint Form
C: Poster

Distribution:
All Holders of P&P Manuals

Review					
Revise					

Figure 3.3

Sample Patient Complaint Process from Eastern State Hospital: Attachment A (cont.)

NUMBER: [number]

Attachment A

EASTERN STATE HOSPITAL
Williamsburg, Virginia

PATIENT COMPLAINT FORM

ATTENTION: Patient Complaint Liaison		**Phone: [number]**
[office address]		**FAX: [number]**
Patient's Name:		**Date:**
Building	**Ward:**	**Date of Complaint**

Figure 3.3

Sample Patient Complaint Process from Eastern State Hospital: Attachment B (cont.)

Comp No. _____ Patient Name: ______________________ File No. ______________________

Building _____ Ward: _________ Date of Complaint: _____________

Nature of Complaint:

____
____
____
____

Category of Complaint ______________________ Sub-Cat: ______________________

Date Received: _________________________ Date Patient Consulted: _________________________

Departments or Personnel Conferred with:

____
____
____
____

Proposed Resolution

____
____
____
____

Date Resolution Discussed with Patient: ________ Date Resolved: ___________

Patient Comments:

____
____
____
____

Patient agrees to resolution: YES NO Patient Signature (optional):

____

30-day follow-up:

____
____
____
____

Patient Complaint Liaison Signature: __________________________ Date Signed: _______________

cc: Hospital Director
Director, QM
Filc

Subject to the Privacy Act of 1974. Unauthorized disclosure is prohibited.

Figure 3.3

Sample Poster Displayed for Staff: Attachment C (cont.)

Eastern State Hospital in cooperation with the Office of Human Rights in an effort to promote patient's rights has developed an internal complaint process.

- Anyone who believes that a provider has violated an individual's rights may report the alleged violation.

- The attempt to resolve the complaint shall be immediate. If the complaint is not resolved to the individual's or legally authorized representative's satisfaction, within five (5) working days, the complaint will be forwarded to the Human Rights Advocate Office.

- If the complaint is not resolved to the individual's or legally authorized representative's satisfaction, the Human Rights Advocate Office will be notified.

- The individual or the legally authorized representative may contact the Office of Human Rights at anytime.

If you have a complaint, contact the Patient Complaint Liaison in Building [number] at [telephone number] or fax your complaint form to [fax number].

CHAPTER 4

Processing the Complaint and Preparing to Respond

CHAPTER 4

Processing the Complaint and Preparing to Respond

Introduction

Patient relations positions at hospitals are becoming more important due to the new focus on identifying opportunities for performance improvement and increasing patient satisfaction scores for public reporting. This is one of the major goals for the patient relations staff. And to succeed, patient relations staff must have the authority to address the complaints so they can advocate for the patient and effect change.

Authority to transform complaints into useful feedback is essential or complaints become a meaningless hassle for management. The goal should not be to stop complaints; rather it should be to use them effectively. The goal is to learn what your organization could do better each time, and to learn why patients get upset, especially in cases when your employees believe they did nothing wrong.

How can you use this information?

Share it with your departments. Incorporate the letters as training handouts to give the patient's perspective. Show all employees the letter in Figure 4.2. Build the tips from St. Vincent Charity Hospital (below) into orientation; have your executives reinforce your commitment to service recovery and complaint management by attending and speaking at this orientation. And help all your caregivers and administrative personnel understand that the more satisfied the patient is, the more likely they will comply with treatment regimens and refer others to your institution. It's not just good business; it's good health care.

St. Vincent Charity Hospital in Cleveland, Ohio, manages complaints using the following process:

Step 1: The patient representative (also known as the patient advocate or patient relations manager) talks to dissatisfied patients or families and friends as soon as possible after a complaint is lodged, or as soon as they learn that a patient is dissatisfied.

Step 2: Patient representative takes care of the concern immediately, if the problem can be resolved easily. If it requires an investigation, then set a goal to completely resolve the issue within 10 business days or less.

Step 3: Use scripting when talking to the patient's family or friend to help you collect the important information you need to resolve the concern or complaint (see the 5-step sample script process in Figure 4.6). Once you complete the initial conversation with the family or friend—and document the details on the scripting form—urge physicians and caregivers to join you in a private conference to discuss the issue. Set up this meeting while the patient is still at the hospital. If the patient was discharged, try to set up a conference when all parties can attend, in person. This meeting helps lower risk by diffusing the situation before it escalates into a lawsuit.

TIP: Disgruntled families want to know that you are taking their issues seriously and that you are doing something about them. Most litigation involves poor communication among caregivers, physicians, and the family. The faster you intervene and allow families to discuss their concerns with caregivers, the more likely the patient will leave with a positive impression of your facility.

Step 4: To judge your success, do what many hospitals such as Waterbury (Connecticut) Hospital and St. Vincent Charity Hospital do: look at your hospital's scores from Press Ganey, the firm that helps health care providers measure patient satisfaction.

Step 5: Look at trends in the patient complaint log and set goals to train workers on how to prevent these complaints.

Getting the caregivers to support you in resolving complaints

It's not easy encouraging and soliciting complaints. And it's perhaps harder to get employees to report what they hear, for fear the hospital could reprimand them. Here are some tips to help you with these challenges:

Step 1: Set up a meeting with each department so that all of your caregivers are very familiar with your hospital's patient representative or patient and family services advocate. This job title will vary by organization, for example, at some facilities, the patient relations manager handles this function. If you don't have an employee to serve as a patient advocate, hire one immediately, but don't appoint the risk manager to this function. Risk management directors have a critical role in the complaint management process (see Figure 4.7 for a suggested flow chart), but their role is different than the patient advocate's.

When meeting with caregivers, the patient representative should share the internal phone number that workers may call to report complaints. Also, share the location of the patient representative's office. Tell workers that it's critical for them to report patient concerns immediately so that the patient representative can help the worker and the patient solve the problem, prevent unproductive communication, and improve future service.

Also reinforce that it's critical for the worker to attempt to resolve or at least listen to the complaint while waiting for the patient representative to arrive. Teach workers how to handle difficult situation and difficult people. For example, hand out the "Hostility Curve," which workers can use as a guide to help them understand the patient's anger and what they need. See Chapter 11, "Replies: Dealing with difficult situations, difficult people and patient errors," for more information about how to handle difficult people and difficult situations.

Step 2: Give them other tools to fix the everyday problems, things like the following:

- Delay in getting an x-ray interpreted
- A longer-than-expected wait in the ED
- A room not as clean as it ought to be
- An employee who treats a patient with disrespect or rudeness

Set an institutional policy allowing caregivers to purchase something from the gift shop. Set some dollar limit guidelines. At St. Vincent Charity Hospital, the risk management department encourages caregivers to attempt to resolve the complaints first before purchasing the gift. Never fall back on the gift as the resolution. The gift should only be a kind of peace offering, an apology. This is the least you can do for the patient who is willing to complain and give you tangible evidence about your services. Now that's a gift!

Step 3: Put the number up on a bulletin board in each patient's room and in a brochure that patients should receive at the beginning of their hospital stay.

Step 4: Set up a meeting to train the medical records department on when and why to contact both the patient representative and the risk management department. At St. Vincent Charity Hospital, medical records must call the risk department each time a patient says they are upset with their care, or when they want to send something to an attorney.

Step 5: Make sure all new employees understand the process for handling complaints—and why—by educating them during orientation.

Step 6: Urge volunteers and people from pastoral care who visit the patients to find out how their stay is going and whether there is anything they can do for them.

Educating staff about the complaint management process

When holding a training session on the complaint management process, focus on helping your employees understand the three basic steps in a complaint management process:

1. Intake (receive complaint)
2. Investigate
3. Respond

Figure 4.1 **Summary of Complaint Resolution Process**

Following is a general guide for patient advocates and patient relations directors on how they can simplify the complaint management process and keep the CEO informed about progress in this area.

Intake

- Receive complaint and send an acknowledgement letter (within three business days).
- Summarize issues and outline action steps and a realistic timeframe to respond.
- Complete a data form (see sample).
- Enter into a database.

Key points: always acknowledge their concerns, apologize for their experience and set appropriate expectations for follow up.

Investigate

- Gather pertinent information (i.e., medical record, itemized billing statement)
- Discuss with manager how the event occurred from the employee point of view.
- Identify key managers and staff involved and organize a meeting.
- Distribute the complaint to the identified group.
- Facilitate the meeting, focus on current process and potential improvements, agree on next steps and timeframe for follow up.

Key points: focus on process and remove personal blame and defensive behaviors by explaining that the goal is to find a way to not let this happen to other patients.

Respond

- Respond to the complainant and explain what actions will take place to improve the situation.
- Report at least quarterly to management.

Key points: convey the hospital's concern with their issue and thank them for taking the time to provide feedback.

How much effort is put into each of these three areas depends on the severity and complexity of the complaint. For example, the action taken regarding a security guard who had a poor attitude will be different from the breech of privacy or confidentiality.

The process needs to be simple and supported by leadership. Too often the patient relations function is to receive and pass the complaint to the department involved. It is more effective if the patient relations staff have the authority to address the issues directly and assist management the with performance and service improvement projects in response to complaints.

Figure 4.2

Sample Patient Complaint

Note: This is an actual letter from a patient that was hand-delivered to the hospital's information desk. It illustrates what can happen when no one takes responsibility for a patient's concern. It also shows how patients are becoming savvier in documenting each conversation they have with health care providers, and how this documentation could one day be used in court.

TIP: Use this as a cautionary letter and as a training tool to educate all of your health care staff—clinical and administrative—about the importance of follow-through and service.

To whom it may concern:

On February______, I came to ______Hospital for a CAT-scan for kidney stones. The purpose of this was six months ago my doctor found that I had 18 stones and am currently undergoing treatment to get rid of the stones and prevent others from forming. The scan on February______ was to find out the progress of the treatment and to plan for future treatment. Since I still pass stones and have considerable pain, it is important that if the current treatment is not working my doctor needs to take another course of treatment.

Here is the current problem. February______was over a month ago or 33 days ago. My doctor has asked me for the results of the scan several times and when I had to see him on March______ for pain from current stones passing he informed me that his office had called the hospital and was told that the CAT scan was never done! I called Friday morning, March ______and was told by a woman in radiology that the report was there but had never been written up and she was going to find out why it wasn't written up and calls me back within an hour (that was 10:07 am).

At 3:30 pm I called my doctor after not hearing anything from the hospital and was told that there was still no report. I then called your hospital back and was assured I would get a return call. At 4:52 pm I got a call from ______ who assured me he would call my doctor. He called me back in 10 minutes and informed me that my doctor's office was closed and that he would see to it that my doctor had the report this morning and he took my doctor's phone number and fax number.

At 11:55 today, March______ I called my doctor to again find out there is still no report. My doctor is assuming I never had the scan done and am only attempting to get pain medicine.

Figure 4.2

Sample Patient Complaint (cont.)

I have called the hospital four times today and had my call answered by a rude operator who I was just trying to get to direct me to someone who would help me. Instead, she only wanted to make a point of telling me she just answered phones and transfer me to lines that just rang 20 times.

So since my doctor cannot get a report from something that was done well over a month ago, I have contacted my insurance company and told them NOT TO PAY YOU FOR THE CAT scan! My doctor is going to issue a new order for a CAT scan and I will take my business to another hospital.

This is to serve as notice that if you attempt to collect for this CAT scan, I will have my attorney issue a lawsuit for harassment and anything else he can get. This is the sorriest excuse I have ever seen for medical service. Eight months ago my wife was told that she had cancer. Trusting ______ Hospital we brought her there for her biopsy. We were told the results would take 2 to 3 days and my family came in from out of state to be with us since we were told that the cancer was on her lungs, kidneys spleen and liver. The results should have been in on the following Monday at the latest and again on the following Tuesday we were told "the results had not been typed up." I had to throw a fit in order to get the results; we were left to wonder how much time she had left and no one cared. As it turned out she did not have cancer but you put us and a lot of family members through a lot of grief because of the total laziness of the radiology department.

I know it is total laziness because I have sat in that department and listened to employees on the phone talking and gossiping about coworkers but they can't type a report and get it to the doctors!

If I am contacted for payment of the CAT scan done on February______ I assure you I will sue you for everything I can get for what is nothing short of failure to perform a service. I have never sued or wanted to sue anyone for anything but after the useless excuse for the way your hospital has performed you deserve it.

[Name of patient]
[Contact Information]

Intake: Receiving, categorizing and tracking complaints

The intake step will categorize the complaint to determine how patient relations will handle it. Some are resolved quickly and require minimal intervention and follow up and others will offer an opportunity for improvement. Categorize them into a broad "issue type" to assist in the tracking of the information:

- System-wide issue
- Quality/Safety issue
- Staff/customer service issue

System-wide issues involve situations that cross over many departments. Examples include an outdated registration system, an unresponsiveness patient transporter system, or the lack of handicap parking. These worthwhile projects must involve a dedicated team, a formal process improvement facilitator, and resources to respond to the outcome. Many resources are available for formal process improvement initiatives.

Figure 4.3

Sample of Intake Data Form

Date Reported _____ / _____ / _____ Patient Name _______________________________

Complainant Name ____________________ Relation to patient ______________________

Telephone ( ) ______ - __________ Date of Service _____ / _____ / _____

Medical Record # _______________ ACCT# __________________

Department in Concern:_______________

Description of Concern:

____

Complaint Category:

❑ **Customer Service** ❑ **Staff** ❑ **Safety** ❑ **Billing** ❑ **Other**

__Not helpful	__Inaccurate info	__Privacy/confidentiality
__Physician issue	__Billing-question	__Wait time
__Medication issue	__Lost item	__Cleanliness
__Bill-error	Responsiveness	__Inaccurate info/error
__General question	__Other staff issue	__Repeated attempts to resolve
__Poor attitude	__Poor coordination	__Inappropriate behavior
__Nursing issue	__Parking	

Action required? ___ Yes ___ No

Actions taken:

____

Resolved? ___ Yes ___ No

Type of service recovery ______________________________ $ __________

Date resolved _____ / _____ / _____

Investigate: Researching the complaint and determining whether intervention is required

The severity of a quality/safety issue will dictate which department is most appropriate to handle the complaint. Patient relations staff may become involved to assist in the investigation, but the qualifications of a risk/quality management department, peer review committee or nursing director may be necessary.

Patient relations staff best handles issues that relate to complaints of employee attitude or customer service inefficiencies. During the investigation step of these complaints, the patient relations staff remains a neutral party. After the investigation step, it is determined the level, if any, of intervention. Some complaints may not require any action, some require an employee's behavior to be addressed, and others warrant an ad hoc group to gather and discuss what happened and how it could have been a better experience for the patient or family member.

When the complaint does warrant an ad hoc group, you need to prepare for the meeting. Identify the key issues from the complaint that need to be discussed and group similar issues together and use this as the agenda. At the meeting the group can review the issues by process and remove defensive behavior in response to the complaint. Examples of these issues include

- poor coordination within a process or between departments
- poor attitude displayed by employee(s)
- breech of privacy/confidentiality perceived by patient
- lack of responsiveness to patient's needs and concerns

Creating improvements based on complaints is difficult in most organizations. Managers are protective over their department and have difficulty with an "outsider" trying to fix problems; and employees sometimes are not aware of how they are perceived by the patient and family members and they become defensive to criticism. The following are examples of the most common challenges to overcome in process and service improvement:

- Defensive behavior—blame the complainer
- Resistance to change
- Not accepting that the problem exists
- Lack of skills

Although it cannot be the responsibility of patient relations to solve these problems, it is essential to have the authority and organizational support to address these challenges. Training and education for staff regarding the proper way to handle and respond to complaints as well as customer service training begins to provide the skills necessary to resolve problems sooner and reduces the severity of complaints.

Response: Documenting the complaint and replying to the complainant

Responding to complaints is a blend of skill and finesse. The investigation step should have organized and addressed the issues that need to be mentioned in the response letter. Some tips regarding your response letter include the following:

- Use a friendly yet professional tone
- Remove health care language that may not be understood by the general public.
- Directly address the issue(s) that were raised—do not ignore the difficult ones
- Never put the blame on the complainant for the incidence
- Always encourage the complainant to contact you with more questions
- Always end with appreciation for their feedback

The person who sent the complaint letter typically is not expecting you to "fix the problem" but they want to know that an honest effort was made for some improvement to occur or a behavior to be addressed. Your response should demonstrate that you took the complaint seriously and that you followed through based on their feedback.

It is not the role of the patient relations staff to judge whether a complaint is true or false. It is the responsibility of the patient relations staff to educate hospital employees that the perception of the patient and family members are important, valued, and never judged.

Figure 4.4 Key Points to Remember When Responding to Complaints

- Listen carefully to the complaint.
- Always be on the lookout for system's issues.
- Do a thorough investigation.
- Recruit appropriate caregivers to analyze the system and develop an action plan.
- Follow up to ensure the action plan is carried out.
- Include administration when necessary.
- Document the process according to the institution's PI policy.
- Patient complaints are your friend. They can lead to performance improvement, increased patient safety, and satisfied customers.

Performance improvement and patient complaints

Meeting with dissatisfied patients to improve performance

In response to a patient's complaint, a Midwestern hospital requested that the complainant meet with the nurse managers and risk managers to discuss the events and which parts were problems. Even though the issue centered on a different hospital, the hospital planned to find ways to improve their own performance and ensure they did not create dissatisfaction. This is an excellent example of how to find a creative way to learn from patient complaints and the following letter is a good example of how to concisely validate the complaint and explain the process.

Issue: Patient transfer

[Date]

[Name]
[Address]

Dear ___________ ,

Thank you again for taking time to discuss your concerns regarding the events surrounding Mr. [name]'s transfer. I was happy to hear the good report on his progress.

After I spoke with you, I discussed the incident again with the supervisors. Please be assured that we have reviewed this matter with all concerned. We realize that we will never be able to control how another hospital will respond (luckily, the situation is rare). However, we did use the event as an opportunity to review how to respond to similar situations, and deliver good customer service.

Our nursing department is very interested in pursuing your ideas of improving our processes. I mentioned to them that your job is related to customer service. If you would be willing, we would like to schedule a meeting at your convenience with the nurse managers involved and me. I would like them to have the chance to listen you your perceptions of the event and more importantly be able to hear how you feel we may be able to change and improve this part of our service.

I realize this is not a typical customer service response, but you are not just a typical customer. Perhaps we may discover a new way to look at things and feel creative about problem solving.

You have provided us with very useful suggestions and information. Thank you for bringing this to our attention. Your opinion about our hospital, staff and the care you receive here is extremely valuable to us. We seem pretty convinced that meeting with you would be beneficial to us. If you feel like you are able to do this, please, call me at [telephone number].

Very Sincerely,

[Name]
[Title]

Case studies demonstrate how patient complaints play a leading role in performance improvement

St. Vincent Charity Hospital in Cleveland, Ohio, assembled a team of nurses, secretaries, aides and managers to discuss one patient's complaint that a nurse never followed-up with her after responding to her call bell at the desk.

During their investigation, the team uncovered several pitfalls. For example, the secretary did not communicate directly with the nurse, the nurse did not hear the page, and the staff did not know whether someone had already answered the call. To remedy the situation, the team decided to directly page the nurse or aide via a beeper that would indicate which patient needed assistance. The idea was taken to administration and the budget was approved for the pagers. The nurses conducted a trial for one month and found that the patient satisfaction scores increased and call lights were answered in a timely manner.

Patient complaints play a leading role in performance improvement. Although not every complaint results in performance improvement, a trend of similar complaints can. They therefore developed an approach to process the complaints. First, they categorized the complaint in order to track it, then they followed these steps:

- Carefully listen to the complaint
- Be objective and supportive
- Verify key issues with the patient/family member
- Set a time to get back to them if the complaint requires investigation
- Investigate the issues with all those who were involved if the complaint warrants it

If the investigation identifies a process issue do the following:

- Work with key people to identify areas for improvement
- Create an action plan
- Implement the plan
- Evaluate the effectiveness with quality indicators
- Document per the institution's performance improvement policy

Following are eight examples of various types of complaints and how the hospital handled them. The method used to resolve the issues may vary. It is therefore important to look closer at each type of complaint and show how it can lead to change. See also the other chapters in this book for sample letters.

Minimizing risk after a patient develops an ulcer—nursing issue

Medical records notified the risk management department that a patient's wife requested a copy of her husband's medical records. While doing so, she informed them that her husband was transferred to a rehabilitation hospital where they found an ulcer on his heel. She stated that the caregivers there told her that it was due to poor care and it would surely delay his physical therapy.

The risk manager called the wife and inquired further about her complaints. After listening carefully to her and clarifying the issues, he started an investigation. The first step was to review the medical records.

The records indicated that Mr. X was a morbidly obese patient who was admitted to the hospital for knee replacement surgery. Following surgery, he was placed in a regular bed with traction bars and a trapeze. TED hose were applied bilaterally and a continuous positive motion machine was used for approximately five hours daily to the surgical leg. Mr. X complained of pain in his foot a few days after surgery and was found to have a large blister to the heel. A dry sterile dressing was applied to the heel, however a physician did not look at the heel for several days. The area turned into an ulcer, requiring medications and treatments for over two months.

After discussing the case with the caregivers, several systems issues were identified.

1. TED hose were removed, but nobody assessed the heels.

2. Mr. X was tall and his feet hit the footboard.

3. Heel pads are not routinely used on knee replacement patients and the current product does not keep pressure off the heel.

4. The blister was not communicated between caregivers and physicians.

The caregivers devised and implemented the following action plan:

1. Nursing will inspect the heels every shift.

2. Nursing staff will ask the patient every shift if they are having pain in the heels.

3. A section was added to the nursing shift assessment to document the condition of the heels.

4. New products were reviewed and tested in a trial to replace the foam heel pads.

5. Tall patients will automatically be put into a longer bed to decrease pressure to the heels.

6. Patients are educated to inform the physician of any problems or concerns in addition to telling the nurse.

In this case, a family conference with physicians and caregivers was held to allow the family to voice their concerns. The family was satisfied with the answers and the action plans; no further follow up was necessary. It is important to note that medical records needs to be on the alert for any potential claims and report them immediately to the risk manager for follow up. Early intervention is essential to resolve issues before they turn into litigation.

Physicians not following procedure—physician issue

Complaints can surface in the most unexpected places, for instance, the medical record. The risk manager came across a nurse's note during a chart review that indicated a patient was upset because he had not seen his surgeon in two days. According to the medical staff policies, the attending physician or his designee must see the patient every day.

Additionally, caregivers were reporting that occasionally surgeons were signing out to the internal medicine physician. However, when they called the internal medicine physician they said they were signed out to the surgeon. It required the caregivers to make several calls to get a physician to manage the patient.

The big question was, "Who is running the ship?" Are the physicians aware of the current medical staff policies? These questions were brought before the surgical committee. After the meeting, it was clear the physicians were not aware of the policy and an action plan was devised that included educating the physicians on the policy and monitoring compliance. Another issue identified was that copies of the bylaws and policies are only given to physicians when they first apply for medical staff privileges. Therefore, they made it a policy to send current copies with the first application and at reappointment.

Preventing medical staff error after complaint—test and treatment issue

A patient called to complain about her bill. She started her story by stating she had surgery last summer and ended up staying three weeks due to complications. According to the patient, she was being fed through a feeding tube when they ran out of her formula and had to substitute another. When her sister came to visit, she found her in a semi-comatose state. The physicians initially thought she had a stroke, but later learned that she suffered a severe hypoglycemic episode because the substituted formula had lower sugar content than the original. Needless to say, the bill was the least of the problems.

The original formula that was ordered was not available. Therefore, the dietitian verbally recommended another product to the Nursing Unit. However, the order that was sent to Dietary from the unit had a totally different product listed. The wrong product was given to the patient for a few days before it was discovered. The physician was unaware of the substitution since nothing was documented on the chart and he was not consulted.

To fix the system, the dietitian drafted a policy indicating steps to take when the formula is out of stock. Instead of recommending the change to nursing, the dietician will now discuss it with the physician. The physician will then write the order and the dietician will document the change in the medical record and notify nursing. By enacting this process, the order will be transcribed by the secretary and sent to dietary and written on the nursing medication record.

Ensuring quality in rooms—a room issue

It is difficult to say that a single complaint in this category led to a performance improvement project. It would be more accurate to say that low Press Ganey scores in this area, as well as complaints from the patients, led to change.

The complaints definitely showed a trend in issues with the cleanliness of the rooms. After careful review and tracking, the hospital changed cleaning companies and hired a new director of environmental services. As a result, patient satisfaction scores have increased and fewer complaints are lodged to the advocate. This area however is continually monitored and tracked for continuous quality improvement.

Improving services for visitors and families

St. Vincent Charity started a program that provides accommodation within the bariatric surgery program for support partners. A few years ago, patients in this program wanted to have someone stay with them the entire time they were in the hospital. However, the visiting policy at the hospital restricted visitors at night and did not have accommodations for rooming-in.

In response to this request, the bariatric surgery program and the surgical unit worked together to allow a support partner to be with the patient throughout his or her stay. A contract was developed outlining the role of the support partner that must be signed by the designated person prior to admission. After surgery, a cot is put in the patient's room for the support partner and they are given an ID badge by security indicating they can visit 24 hours/day.

This program has been very successful and is monitored and re-evaluated on a weekly basis to meet the needs of this population.

Making meals palatable

This is another category where tracking and trending is necessary to make changes. If every complaint resulted in a change, the chef would throw in the apron and the kitchen would be in chaos.

Several complaints were lodged because the patients did not like the taste of the broth that was served on a full liquid diet. According to the dietician, it was an 'acquired' taste since it was low in sodium. It seems as though several people did not acquire the taste. Therefore, the diligent dietary staff taste tested several brands and finally came up with a product that was palatable and acceptable to the patients.

Other patients thought their taste buds were playing tricks on them. They put hot water and tea bags in their cups, but it tasted just like coffee. After a careful investigation, it was discovered that the same cups were being used for both coffee and tea. The cups were retaining the coffee taste and thus making the tea taste like coffee. New cups were ordered in a different color for hot water and the decaffeinated coffee is now identified by a dot that is placed on the lid. The tea drinkers appear to be satisfied at last count. Or, could it mean that only coffee drinkers are being admitted? Further research may be necessary.

Improving discharge planning

Mrs. S was an 80-year-old woman who presented to the emergency department (ED) complaining of shortness of breath and a headache. She is oxygen dependent and has a history of hypertension and chronic lung disease. The nurses noted that she lived alone and her only family was an elderly sister who visited occasionally. Mrs. S also indicated that she recently ran out of her blood pressure medicine and was unable to get to the pharmacy to refill it.

While in the ED, her blood pressure was elevated and her lungs were congested. She was treated with diuretics and discharged with prescriptions and instructions to use her oxygen. A taxi was called to take her home.

In the next two days, Mrs. S came back to the ED twice for similar symptoms. The first time she was treated and released, however the second time she was admitted to the ICU for congestive heart failure and uncontrolled hypertension. She stated she did not take any medications at home because she was unable to get to the pharmacy to fill the prescriptions. In addition, her oxygen tank was empty and the home health care agency was closed for the weekend.

During the admission, her sister was upset because the patient was seen twice in the ED and sent home. She was sure this aggravated her condition and necessitated her ICU admission.

After researching her complaint, it was apparent the patient was sent home without appropriate discharge planning. The physicians and nursing staff did not ask the patient if she was able to get her medications on the way home. They also did not consider the fact that she had to take a taxi home, had no family to help her, and that most pharmacies were closed. They also did not ensure that she had oxygen available at home.

The case managers, pharmacist, and respiratory therapist developed a plan to ensure that all patients have the items necessary for home care. They are now checking with home health to make sure the oxygen tanks are filled and pharmacy now has an after hours plan to get patients a starter pack of medications. This patient could potentially have avoided the second ED visit and admission if she had her medications and oxygen at home. This is not only a cost to the patient but also to the hospital.

Improving the process for transfer fixes a billing issue

A mother called the patient advocate to complain about her son's bill from the ED. Her son had a laceration to his face that required sutures. After waiting two hours, the physician transferred them to another hospital for a plastic surgeon to treat him. She refused to pay the remainder of the bill since he was not treated there.

In order to investigate this complaint, the medical record was reviewed to verify her account of the situation. It was clear from reviewing the record that the physician never filled out a transfer sheet prior to transferring the child. Upon further investigation with the medical director and nurse manager of the ED, several systems issues were identified.

First, the physicians did not think they needed to fill out a transfer sheet if they were going by car. Secondly, they were using a different transfer form than our affiliate. Finally, there were no clear guidelines regarding completion of the transfer form.

As a result, the transfer forms were reviewed and a common form was put into place. A guideline was also developed to indicate when and how to complete a transfer form. Education was provided to all ED staff at both facilities.

This is a perfect example of how a non-related complaint can turn into a performance improvement project. Remember to always keep your eyes and ears open when investigating a complaint. It is amazing what unexpected issues can turn up.

Respecting each patient's individuality—a personal issue

Mr. B was hospitalized with advanced heart disease. In addition, he suffered from end-stage renal disease that required hemodialysis three days per week. During his stay, he suffered a bowel obstruction that necessitated surgery. His condition steadily deteriorated from that day forward. The surgeon met with Mr. B and his wife and they agreed that he would be a comfort care status in the event he arrested.

The following day, Mr. B's cardiologist saw the code status and expressed his dissatisfaction to the family. He insisted, "It's all in God's hands and who are we to get in the way." The family felt compelled to change the code status back to a full code even though it was not what they desired.

During the next few days, the patient and family were very unhappy and finally had the surgeon reverse the code status. A sense of peace and acceptance settled over the couple and he died a few days later.

A hospital chaplain brought the issue to the Ethics Committee for review. It was clear that it was not appropriate for the cardiologist to impose his views on the patient and family and that it went against the core values of the hospital. Therefore, the committee determined that they would provide education to the physicians and caregivers regarding the patient's right to make end of life decisions and respecting their choices.

Protecting patient property and valuables

Mr. G. reports to the nurse that he can't eat dinner because his dentures have vanished. Miss R is complaining that her watch was there a minute ago, but now it is missing. Mrs. T insists that she had her clothes when she came in for surgery, but they are nowhere to be found.

It became apparent after searching for several lost items that an inefficient system was the culprit. The valuables forms were either not filled out completely or were left blank. Many of the lost items were last seen in the same day surgery center where they do not use the valuables form. Nurses were putting items that were left after the patient was transferred or discharged in a storage room on the unit instead of getting them back to the patient. If they weren't claimed they threw them away. Caregivers also complained that the forms were unclear and time-consuming to fill out.

Therefore, a new valuables form was developed and the property policy was revised. Every department responsible for admitting the patient, including same day surgery and ED, was now required to fill out the form and put it on the chart. Education was provided to each department on the new form and policy. Since it was implemented, there has been a significant decrease in lost property complaints. This also represents a huge cost savings for the institution.

Figure 4.5

Patient Representative Complaint Log

CATEGORY	2A	3A	TCU	5B	6A	ICU CSU	CMU CIU	ED	ED/SL	PER	4A	OPS	ACC	OR/RR	TOTAL	%
NURSES																
Friendliness/courtesy/attitude															0	#DIV/0!
Promptness in responding															0	#DIV/0!
Amount of personal attention paid															0	#DIV/0!
Kept me informed															0	#DIV/0!
Have technical skill															0	#DIV/0!
Sensitivity and responsiveness to pain															0	#DIV/0!
PHYSICIAN																
Time spent with you															0	#DIV/0!
Concern for your questions and worries															0	#DIV/0!
How well you were kept informed															0	#DIV/0!
Friendliness/courtesy															0	#DIV/0!
Have technical skill															0	#DIV/0!
How well your pain was controlled															0	#DIV/0!
TEST AND TREATMENTS																
Waiting time															0	#DIV/0!
Concern shown for your comfort															0	#DIV/0!
Explanations about what would happen															0	#DIV/0!
Skill of the person who took blood															0	#DIV/0!
Courtesy of person who took blood															0	#DIV/0!
Skill of person who started the IV															0	#DIV/0!
Courtesy of the person who started IV															0	#DIV/0!
ROOM																
Pleasantness of décor															0	#DIV/0!
Cleanliness															0	#DIV/0!
Courtesy of person who cleaned															0	#DIV/0!
Temperature															0	#DIV/0!
Noise level in and around room															0	#DIV/0!
How well things worked (TV, etc.)															0	#DIV/0!
VISITORS AND FAMILY																
Helpfulness of staff at information desk															0	#DIV/0!
Accommodations and comfort for visitors															0	#DIV/0!
Staff attitude toward your visitors															0	#DIV/0!
Info give to family about pt's condition/tx															0	#DIV/0!
CATEGORY	**2A**	**3A**	**TCU**	**5B**	**6A**	**ICU CSU**	**CMU CIU**	**ED**	**ED/SL**	**PER**	**4A**	**OPS**	**ACC**	**OR/RR**	**TOTAL**	**%**
MEALS																
Special/restricted diet, how well explained															0	#DIV/0!
Temperature of food															0	#DIV/0!
Quality of food															0	#DIV/0!
Courtesy of person serving food															0	#DIV/0!
DISCHARGE																
Extent felt ready to be discharged															0	#DIV/0!
Speed of process															0	#DIV/0!
Instructions/explanations given															0	#DIV/0!
Help with arranging home care service															0	#DIV/0!
PERSONAL ISSUES																
Staff concern for patient privacy															0	#DIV/0!
Sensitivity to emotional/spiritual needs															0	#DIV/0!
Response to concerns/complaints															0	#DIV/0!
Effort to include patient in tx decisions															0	#DIV/0!
Respect for cultural/racial/religious needs															0	#DIV/0!
OVERALL ASSESSMENT & MISC																
How well staff worked together															0	#DIV/0!
Billing Services															0	#DIV/0!
Lost/Broken Property															0	#DIV/0!
Other															0	#DIV/0!
TOTAL	0	0	0	0	0	0	0	0	0	0	0	0	0	0	0	

GRIEVANCES FILED																
SOURCE INFORMATION																
Initial visits by Patient Advocate															0	
Referral/FU															0	
Post Stay Contacts															0	
ADMISSIONS															0	
PATIENT POSITIVES															0	

Figure 4.6 Script for the Risk Management Department

1. Initial Contact (face-to-face)

Hi, Mr./Ms. ________________. My name is ________________ and I am the ________________.
It is my understanding that you wanted to speak to me in regard to ________________ care.

2. Initial Contact (phone)

So that I can understand the situation better, start by giving me your name [and the patient's name that you are referring to].

All right, if you can start from the beginning and tell me what your concerns are.

3. Communicating with unhappy or difficult customers

Use phrases such as:

- Apologies
  - I am/we are so sorry that this happened.
  - Please accept my/our apologies for this.
  - I can see that this has really upset you, and I am very sorry.
  - I am sorry you have had to wait for the doctor/your appointment/me.
  - I wish I could have done something to prevent this from happening, and I am sorry it did.
  - I apologize on behalf of the hospital, for any disturbance that this has caused you.

- Empathy/Sympathy
  - I can see that this has made you very angry.
  - I can understand how you must feel.
  - That must have been a very upsetting experience.
  - I wish I could do more to help you.

- Broken Record
  - I will (call/do X) and then get back to you…
  - I wish I could do more right now, but I can assure you that I will (call or do X) and then contact you right away…
  - As I have tried to reassure you, I promise I will immediately (call or do X) and call you back right away.
  - Again, you have my commitment that I will do as I promised as soon as I leave you.

4. Communicating with upset patient where hospital is at fault

This will vary based on the circumstances and if the patient was injured. This will not occur until the Director of Risk Management has reviewed the complaint.

Figure 4.6 Script for the Risk Management Department (cont.)

- Insurance has paid entire bill

  I can see that this has really upset you, and we're very sorry. However, I have reviewed the medical records and interviewed personnel involved in her care and have found (state findings).

  Our usual method to deal with this type of situation is to waive your deductible or co-pay from your hospital bill. However, the insurance has paid your bill in full. Therefore, how would you like us to resolve this issue for you?

- Insurance has only partially paid the bill

  I can see that this has really upset you Mr./Ms.____________, and we're very sorry. However, I have reviewed the medical records and interviewed personnel involved in his/her care and have found...

  Due to the circumstances, we would be happy to waive any deductibles or co-pays from your hospital bill. I will contact the business office and make arrangements for your bill to be adjusted. In the meantime, if you receive any bills please disregard them.

5. Referring complainant to manager.

- Manager explaining to complainant right to file a grievance:

  "Mr./Ms. _________________, I am sorry but there is nothing more that I can do for you. If you would like, I can have my supervisor call you." If answer is yes, "My supervisor's name is [name]. She will need some time to look into your concerns and will call you within a week."

- If patient expresses that he/she is still not satisfied and want to take this further:

  "Since I have not been able to resolve this matter to your satisfaction, the hospital does have a grievance process. I can have our Patient Representative send you a letter acknowledging your desire to file a grievance if that is what you wish. You may also file a grievance with the state agency: [insert contact information here] "

- If the complainant does not wish to file a grievance:

  "I am sorry that we did not meet your expectations and I do wish you well."

- If the complainant does want to file a grievance:

  "The grievance notification letter will be sent to you within the next working day and a response to the grievance will be provided to you within 40 days from today. If you would like to send your written grievance to the hospital, send it to [specific contact name and address]."

Figure 4.7

Flowchart: Interaction with Patient During Complaint Process

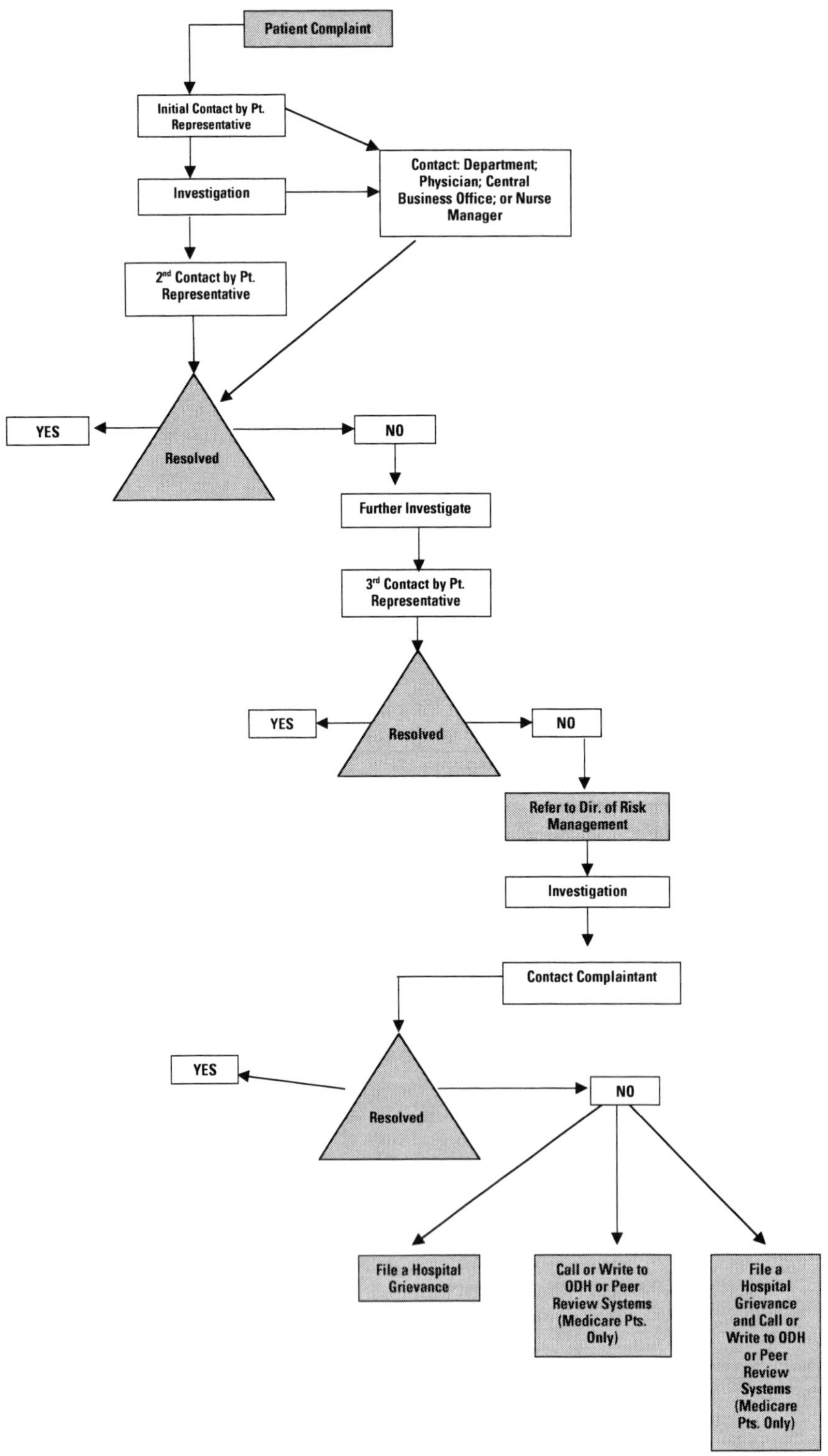

CHAPTER 5

Documenting and Handling Telephone Complaints and On-site Verbal Complaints

Chapter 5

Documenting and Handling Telephone Complaints and On-site Verbal Complaints

There are several issues the patient relations department must consider in order to improve how your facility manages verbal complaints. In some ways, you must become a "complaint recruiter," and encourage the patient community to share all concerns. You must urge staff to report concerns quickly and use your department to help them listen to patients and improve service. Use these seven issues below to improve how your facility handles verbal complaints, and build this information into your orientation and ongoing customer service training with departments. Also see the three letters at the end of this chapter for analysis of real complaints in health care facilities across the country.

Issue 1: Requiring staff to encourage patients and visitors to file a complaint while still in the hospital.

How to implement this approach

Tell staff during training that it's important to handle each "concern" with the same level of care as they would a patient's medical condition. And tell them that as soon as a dissatisfied patient leaves the hospital campus, the odds of losing that patient's business or being sued increase.

Following is how employees should handle specific situations to prevent this:

1. When employees are having difficulty communicating with a patient or family member, or dealing with their concern, they should immediately call the patient representative or another designated person in risk management. Here's an example of a common mistake:

   Patient: "I'm concerned about something that happened with my x-rays. I'm upset about it and need your help."

   Employee: "Sorry, I can't help you. That's not my department. Why don't you try radiology?"

   This example represents the crux of what goes wrong with service. The employee should have asked the patient about what happened and then helped him or her get in touch immediately with the patient representative. Bring employees to the patient representative's office, if possible, or wait with them until the patient representative arrives.

2. Other times, your workers may want to help, but they recognize that the patient does not want to voice their complaint with them. Many people fear retaliation since you are in charge of their medical care. In this case, urge the worker to immediately acknowledge the person's complaint by saying something like the following:

   "I understand you are upset and concerned. Let me help you talk to our patient representative who will listen to your concern."

   Sometimes, that's all the patient wants: to have any hospital representative listen to their concern.

   Unfortunately, too many workers take concerns personally and may never even report the concern. This is when concerns escalate into complaints, or worse.

Issue 2: Handling complaints "at the department level" vs. at the hospital's "patient relations level"

Most hospitals encourage complaint resolution by department. The primary benefit is quick response, as the immediate caregivers probably have more knowledge about the situation that's causing the complaint. This is particularly true of treatment-related concerns.

That said, many departments would prefer to handle the complaint on their own for pride and job security reasons. Local managers do not want to alert the hospital executives that there are issues. This is problematic.

That's why you must build a trust level with departments to let them know that patient relations is here to improve the entire service system in the hospital, not punish one department for every complaint. Complaints are going to happen.

As patient relations managers, educate department heads and nurse managers on your role. Let them know the benefits of your work with a statement like this:

"We aim to fix the process, to improve the service, and to advocate for the patient. And for every concern we handle, we move your department that much closer to being aware of its service challenges and goals."

Tell department heads that patient relations can help each department improve service so that they spend less time addressing complaints and managing patient expectations—and more time focusing on providing the best care possible. Let the complaint-handling experts in patient relations do their part so the clinicians can do theirs.

Patients have the right to ask questions of the nurses and doctors, to ask about advantages and disadvantages of certain tests, treatments, and medications. Remind patients about this right and also let them know they can contact an advocate if they need help advocating for themselves. Patient relations must try to do what it can to collect concerns and complaints, and then help department heads make small changes to prevent them.

Issue 3: Convincing patients that their care won't be jeopardized if they complain on site

If we agree that it's best to hear the complaint while the patient is still in the hospital, then your primary job every day is to build a level of trust with the community. They must know that their complaints will be heard; that they have advocates inside the hospital whose main job is to help them resolve their concerns.

It is very common for older people not to complain because they think their care will be jeopardized. Current methods most hospitals use to let patients know about their rights to complain aren't enough to change their mind. Patient information guides include patient rights, responsibilities, hospital services, and amenities, inform patients on how to complain, but they do little to build the trust.

The patient has the right (by federal law) to file a complaint with the hospital and if they are not satisfied with the outcome, they then possess the right to file a complaint with the state health department. You must include this statement in your admission paperwork, mount it on the walls in patient care areas, or in your patient information guide.

This is typically the only way patients learn how to formally complain. Not that inviting is it? Nor is it completely visible, especially for seniors whose main concern is seeing the nurse or doctor.

Following are some ways to change perceptions and build trust:

- In an ideal world, you could call all discharged patients or at least send them a "thank you for being our patient" letter and include your contact information.
- Include your contact info on your hospital's patient satisfaction surveys that your hospital sends.
- Hand a business card to patients. Departments that tend to generate many complaints—such as emergency and radiology—should also have cards to distribute.

- Post signs on the wall in these and other departments about how patients may file a complaint, where to go or whom to call. Put the patient relations number in large print.

- Use volunteer patient representatives. The patient reps can go into rooms and visit patients and report back to the director. Some hospitals have retirees doing this volunteer work.

- Use your hospital Web site as a means to seek feedback on "concerns" and "complaints." Patients can privately submit a form electronically that will be read by the patient relations department only. Make sure to respond to these complaints—as you would with all verbal and written complaints—as quick as possible. Let patients know on the Internet site that you "appreciate their concern" and will be in touch to discuss it. Establish a response time, like 48 hours as many hospitals have done.

- Contact local reporters at the newspapers and give them the information on how patients can share concerns with the hospital.

Don't hide the fact that your patients can file a complaint. If you can explain the situation and reassure complainants that the hospital takes feedback seriously to improve things, patients and others will release their anger.

TIPS

MAKING EMPLOYEES BETTER REPORTERS

Urge workers to collect the following info when a patient or family member complains to them, especially when the patient representative is busy:

- Patient information
- Date of occurrence
- Who else at the hospital knows about the complaint
- Any quality/safety/risk indications
- Patient's contact information
- Urgency of issue
- Names of other employees involved in the situation
- Patient's and/or family's expectations for follow up

Issue 4: Empowering employees to resolve concerns on the spot

Facilities that require approvals from mid- and upper-management about the handling of each complaint will lose credibility with employees. A "chain in command" arrangement won't work. You cannot have layers of approvals. If you do, complaints will never rise to the top because they will become too much work and follow up. Employees will not make complaint resolution and patient satisfaction a priority if it's too difficult for them.

Solution: Cut out the layers. Empower employees to resolve complaints. Some hospitals have mastered this art, and culled from each complaint an idea or solution to a service issue.

Advise employees in training on how to report complaints. Provide the name and number of one person or department. Health care organizations should not penalize workers for reporting complaints, especially those that the worker caused. Put these rules in writing to reinforce a culture of service recovery.

In training, focus on the positive effects of complaints. Then put this attitude to work, by recognizing employees who have gone out of their way to help patients and families, and those who help patient relations manage and resolve complaints. Recognize employees in public ways, such as through your newsletters or in department meetings. This will help spread awareness of what you do and why it's important.

Issue 5: Educating the front desk

Many complaints come as families are leaving a hospital. A parent may find a receptionist or someone in the Emergency Department and share their experience. Others, still fuming from a bad experience, call the hospital switchboard and sound off to anyone who will listen.

To make sure the receptionists and hospital operators know the role and contact info for patient relations, ask to attend their staff meeting and explain your role and how you help people. Slip in some good customer service skills regarding the types of things you do to respond to the person. Reinforce that you want to help them handle that initial call or customer in-person complaint; but make sure to stress that you and your team are dedicated to handling this task.

Issue 6: Handling concerns from family members when patients are unable to communicate

This happens quite often, especially with mentally ill patients who have died or been transferred to a different facility. Handle these complaints the same as you would all others.

Figure 5.1 **Case Study of In-person Complaint**

Intake

A daughter of a deceased patient came to the hospital a few days after her mother had passed away. She wanted to express her concerns about her late mother's hospital stay. She raised the following issues: a lack of responsiveness by some staff; no one told her about her mother's personal belongings; an unsettled feeling about the hospital.

Investigation

For this visit, I provided a quiet setting to listen to the woman. I took only a few notes in front of her to give her complete attention. Eye contact was important. We exchanged contact information; it did not seem as though the woman wanted much involvement with follow up. She simply wanted to share her concerns and hoped that we would try to improve on our service.

We reviewed the medical record to identify all staff members involved with the mother's care. We reviewed the lengths of time the patient waited during her stay, as well. Then, we held a meeting with the nursing director to talk about staff who may not have been responsive to the patient's needs and how she ought to respond to those employees.

Then we discussed with the unit manager the procedure for unclaimed personal belongings of a deceased patient. Next, we contacted the security department to search for the patient's unclaimed personal belongings.

Respond

We sent a letter to the daughter thanking her for taking the time to provide feedback and asking her if she would like to pick up her mother's personal belongings or have them shipped. We also explained our investigation and how the managers talked to the staff about their unresponsiveness and poor attitude. In this case, we did not need to make any formal service or process improvements since there was no pattern for these complaints on this particular unit.

Source: Waterbury Hospital, Connecticut. Submitted by Cristine Vogel, Manager, Patient Relations.

Since the families or close friends with whom you are dealing are struggling with emotions of death or crisis situations, set limits on what you say over the phone and in person. Consider the family whose father just died in a car accident: What if the family blames the emergency department for the death? This is not uncommon for those dealing with the initial stages of grief. These types of cases carry higher risk for liability because you are often dealing with more tragic circumstances.

Don't offer false hope. Reassure patients that you are here for them and willing to listen. Set up a meeting with your legal counsel and your pastoral care department to discuss the types of phrases and comforting language you can use.

Issue 7: Handling telephone complaints

Many patients and family members who have a complaint with the service at your hospital won't share their experience until after they leave; many people feel more comfortable sending an e-mail or calling the hospital.

For those with the most serious complaints, expect a phone call on the day or week the patient is discharged. Take these complaints very seriously and handle with extreme care. The reason: Patients and families in these circumstances typically leave the hospital upset, mull over their experience, and then call. This means their complaint is legitimate, even if you later determine that the hospital staff did nothing legally or medically wrong.

It's very difficult to satisfy an upset person over the phone. It takes a patient tone and a helpful approach. Make sure your staff know to forward these calls directly to the patient relations line.

Here are some tips for dealing with people who call in their concern or complaint:

- Never put these people on hold.
- If they leave a voicemail, call back as soon as you receive the message
- If they are not in when you return their call, leave a brief message with a sincere tone and tell them that you "appreciate their call and want very much to talk to them." Give them a backup number, such as cell, if you have one.

Here are some reminders to keep in mind—consider posting them by your phone—for the actual phone conversation:

- Listen, do not interrupt.
- Be compassionate, not defensive.
- Acknowledge the person's unhappiness and express understanding about their experience—but do not agree with the situation.
- Write down pertinent details. This is an important step as miscommunication often occurs at this point. It's critical to get the correct concern on paper; this will help you investigate.
- Repeat your interpretation of the issues for clarification purposes.
- Explain the next steps that will occur.
- Set a realistic date for follow up, if necessary.
- Investigate or report the complaint to the patient relations department.
- Respond with resolution.

When properly handled, you can use telephone complaints to diffuse a potentially litigious situation and help your facility improve service. And as with all complaint management, the key is to deliver on your promise and follow up with the patient when you say you will.

Verbal and telephone complaints—sample letters and memos

Below are two letters and a memorandum regarding verbal and telephone complaints from patients to hospitals.

1. The memo

This does a good job of laying out the facts and outlining the people involved, but there are some issues to watch for. Under "Investigative Findings," the hospital should have been more careful about assuming the daughter knew about how to contact patient relations. Rethink using a statement like this in #5: "*The patient's daughter never contacted the patient relations office regarding her concerns during her mother's hospitalization.*"

This finding is somewhat presumptive. Some patients and family members don't feel comfortable making complaints on-site; others aren't given the proper information, or the patient relations department may not be visible.

Complaint:
The Commonwealth of Virginia, Department of Health, Center for Quality Health Care Service and Consumer Protection, received a verbal complaint from [complainant name], the daughter of patient, [patient name]. The Hospital was requested to submit a written response to the complainant and to send a copy of the response within forty-five days to the Complaint Supervisor at the aforementioned Agency at the Department of Health.

Summary of the issues that were reported:
"The complainant, [name], stated that her mother, [name], who was admitted to [name] Hospital on [date], received unacceptable care. The complainant stated that her mother's calls for help were not answered, that her mother had numerous unnecessary tests and that her mother developed a bedsore because hospital staff did not turn her regularly. The complainant also stated that her mother was discharged without receiving physical therapy."

I attempted to call the patient's daughter for further details and received a call back from the Department of Health stating that the complainant had noted the call from the Hospital via her caller ID and did not wish to discuss this with anyone from [name] Hospital.

Investigative findings per review of medical record and interviews with all departments involved:

1. Patient was being seen and followed by a registered dietician, and was also receiving Total Parenteral Nutrition via IV.

2. Patient was being attended by a wound care nurse, who documented that patient told her "I don't like being on my side, so I roll onto my back when the nurses leave the room".

3. Physical therapy was ordered for endurance. Eighteen visits by a physical therapist were documented in the patient's record. One note indicated that the patient's daughter was in the room when the therapist visited. It was further noted that the patient refused therapy numerous times, saying that she was too weak or too tired.

4. The patient had multiple, complex medical problems and the attending physician called in appropriate consultants for her problems.

5. The patient's daughter never contacted the patient relations office regarding her concerns during her mother's hospitalization.

2. Letter 1: Sincere apology example

If you are writing a letter in follow up to a productive conversation with a patient, reinforce, as the writer has done, your institution's sincere apology. Express appreciation for the time the patient spent with you over the phone. Remember, the patient doesn't have to share the complaint. Apologies, like those in these letters, also work well to express compassion, but not admit guilt. There's a fine balance and these letters meet it.

[Date]

[Name]
[Address]

Dear______________,

Thank you so much for taking the time to call and speak with me regarding your recent visit to the emergency room at [name] Hospital. Please be assured that we have taken your concerns very seriously.

Your concern about the treatment you received from the physician has been shared with both the director and the medical director of the emergency department. While there are certain tests that must be run when you present with certain symptoms, we are very sorry that there was such poor communication. It is never our goal to treat any patient in a condescending or rude manner. Please accept our apology for this very negative experience.

We do strive for excellence in patient care and customer service. Feedback such as yours is very helpful as we strive to improve the services that we offer. Thank you for giving us a chance to review our performance. If there if anything further that I may assist you with please feel free to call me at [telephone number].

Sincerely,

[Name]
[Title]

CC: [Name(s) and Title(s)]

3. Letter 2: Unable to reach complainant

This letter works well because it's not defensive. Use this simple 3-step strategy for writing letters after you've tried to reach a patient, but have no luck or meet resistance:

1. Start with the apology
2. Blend in the facts only—not your opinion—about your attempt to reach them. Don't dwell on this, or blame the patient. Make your language fact-focused. For example, when stating that a patient did not return a call or chose not to discuss the situation over the phone, never start the sentence with the word "But." This is a defensive word. Simply state the fact the way the writer did in the first sentence in the second paragraph of the final letter.
3. Quickly give the patient or family member the opportunity to call anytime.

[Date]

[Name]
[Address]

Dear___________,

Thank you sharing information about your recent experience at [name] Hospital. We sincerely regret our service did not meet your expectations. In order for us to make corrective changes and improvements we have tried to call your home in an attempt to gather details about the specific aspects of your care that were dissatisfying.

You did not want to discuss your concerns with us. However, if you should change your mind please feel free to contact me at [telephone number] or our Vice President of Patient Services, [Name], at [telephone number].

We want to be your health care system of choice. In the future we look forward to continuing to serve you and your family with the highest possible quality of care.

Sincerely,

[Name]
[Title]

Cc: [Name], Vice President of Patient Services
Master File OPT Support Services

SECTION II

HOW TO RESPOND TO TYPICAL GRIEVANCES

SECTION II CONTENTS

CHAPTER 6

Initial Replies: Responding to the First Communication

Chapter 6

Initial Replies: Responding to the First Communication

Introduction

How you receive a complaint varies. A patient may leave a note in his room when upon discharge, sometimes she may pass a note to a nurse, other patients may hand-deliver a letter, still others may send it by mail, some even by return receipt. No matter which method, in the end, you have in your hand written proof of a dissatisfied patient.

Many times patients take initiative and provide feedback on their own. However, other times, you may have to try to get the feedback. Soliciting feedback through patient satisfaction surveys is an excellent way to learn what patients liked—and didn't like—about their time in your facility. Surveys don't need to be long; some may be a few short, yet pertinent, questions that you can fit on a postcard. It is important, however, to ensure that you follow-up with patients who responded. Some hospitals also invite some patients to "brown bag roundtable" lunches to provide face-to-face feedback.

Your hospital—and likely other organizations that affect your hospital such as the state and accreditors—will have suggestions, requirements and guidelines for how you must address patient grievances. Make sure to review the information in Section I to learn about legal requirements, HIPAA, and other important information you need to know before addressing a patient complaint.

This chapter contains sample letters that are the first reply to a patient complaint.

Dissatisfied patients respond to patient satisfaction survey

Analysis: The following two letters are replies to patient satisfaction surveys—and clearly are not on the high end of satisfied. The complaints were sent to the emergency department manager who is a registered nurse. The strength of these letters are how they are short and to the point. They are reassuring and validating. However, they do offer an apology in a way that might make the facility vulnerable. Keep in mind that it is important to apologize for how the patient perceived his or her care, rather than admitting wrongdoing. A better apology in the first case might be, "Please accept our sincerest apology that our care did not meet your expectations; we are sorry that you did not feel you were treated in a timely manner."

Issue: Care was not timely

[Date]

[Name]
[Address]

Dear Ms. ______,

Thank you for taking the time to respond to our Patient Satisfaction Survey regarding your visit to our emergency department on [Date]. We appreciate feedback because it enables us to improve our service and care of our patients and their families at [Name of organization]. Exceptional quality and service to all of our patients and their families is our highest priority.

Please accept our sincere apology for the inconvenience of not treating you in a timely manner. This is one aspect of care we are diligently working to improve, in spite of the national trend of increased overcrowding of emergency rooms.

Again, thank you for taking the time to inform us of your concerns and offering us your feedback. Should you have additional concerns or questions, please feel free to contact me at any time at [number and or e-mail].

Sincerely,

[Name]
[Title]

Issue: Patient did not receive clear discharge instructions

[Date]

[Name]
[Address]

Dear Ms. ______:

Thank you for taking the time to respond to our Patient Satisfaction Survey regarding your visit to our emergency department on [Date]. We appreciate feedback because it enables us to improve our service and care of our patients and their families at [Name of organization]. Exceptional quality and service to all of our patients and their families is our highest priority.

Please accept our sincere apology for the inconvenience of not receiving clear discharge instructions from our facility. We are currently in the process of identifying and making the necessary changes to our computerized discharge information system, in order to prevent this problem from occurring in the future. Please be assured that your response will be handled confidentially and our management team will take corrective action. Exceptional quality and service to each of our patients is our highest priority.

Again, thank you for taking the time to inform us of your concerns and offering us your feedback. Should you have additional concerns or questions, please feel free to contact me at any time at [number and/or e-mail].

Sincerely,

[Name]
[Title]

Written complaints sent by mail

Issue: Patient received poor care in emergency room

Analysis: This letter is sent from the Senior Vice President of Medical Staff Affairs. The strength here is level of detail: explanation of policy, how this incident is inconsistent with it and the process this complaint will follow (mainly second paragraph). The statement in third paragraph is a good statement of goal/mission. The last paragraph is a nice way to wrap up.

[Date]

[Name]
[Address]

Dear ____________,

Thank you for taking time to provide feedback regarding your recent care at [Name of organization]. Please accept my sincere apology for our failure to meet expectations during your emergency room visit in [date] and hospitalization in [date].

The events you described are not consistent with [Name of organization] values and standards for performance. The [Name of organization] Peer Review Committee will review your letter and chart. Any issues identified by that committee will be addressed with the physicians involved.

At [Name of organization], we encourage and value feedback from our patients and their families. Our goal is for each patient to have a positive experience with our services. We appreciate the opportunities to improve our processes and services. Should you have any further questions or would like to discuss specific issues that caused you concern, please contact our Director of Quality Management, [name] at [telephone and/or e-mail].

Again, I apologize for your recent experience. If you or a member of your family has a future need for health care services, I would like [Name of organization] to be your provider of choice.

Sincerely,

[Name]
[Title]

Issue: Dispute about billing

Analysis: The Director of Quality/Care Management sent this letter. This response could easily be to a verbal complaint as well as written. The weakness of this letter is that it is very vague about the billing issue. Without breaching privacy or legal issues, it is possible to provide slightly more detail that will help you in case you (or someone else) need to reference this letter to recall the situation. The strength of this letter is how it discusses the process and validates the issue, as well as reassuring the patient about privacy. The letter also contains a carbon copy name. One name is reasonable. Keep in mind it can undermine your word as the hospital's representative if the cc list is too long.

[Date]

[Name]
[Address]

Dear _____________,

CONFIDENTIAL

[Name of employee] has shared your concerns regarding your recent emergency department visit. Thank you for taking time to bring your billing issues to our attention.

We collect this information and regularly discuss the issues with the corresponding service departments in order to keep our charges consistent with billing practices in our area, and the law. Although your personal identity is protected in this process, we will review your concerns within a group of similar concerns.

We are always looking for creative ways to deliver better service to our customers in more efficient and cost-effective ways. The information you have provided is a valuable tool in that process.

Again, thank you for bringing this to our attention. Your opinions about our hospital, staff and the care you receive here is extremely valuable to us. If ever I can be of any help to you, or if you feel this matter warrants further discussion, please feel free to contact me at [telephone number and/or e-mail].

Very Sincerely,

[Name]
[Title]

CHAPTER 7

Follow-up Replies: Responding Throughout the Process and Communicating the Status of the Investigation

Chapter 7

Follow-up Replies: Responding Throughout the Process and Communicating the Status of the Investigation

Why it is important to communicate with dissatisfied patients throughout the process

Business communication 101: The patient thinks her complaint is the only one. And so this must be how your patient relations team treats each person's case. For complaints that you cannot resolve immediately with a phone call and a letter, make a habit of staying in touch. See the letters in the section, "Communicating the status of the investigation" for real examples. Send these "updates" as your peers have done here to keep the family or patient posted on the progress of your investigation. This will reassure people that your hospital is taking their complaint seriously and prevent the issue from escalating. If you forget to do this, the complaint becomes idle and the patient may take feel betrayed and consider a suit.

Failing to follow up with someone who complained is one of the major reasons hospitals are sued. There are numerous cases of family members who make repeated verbal and written complaints, only to never hear from the hospital. This means the process broke down. To avoid this, instruct all employees who receive a verbal or written complaint or concern from a patient or family member to document the specifics and then share them with the patient relations department.

The letters in this section illustrate the importance of follow up: how to do it well, what to avoid, and what your peers say in their responses.

Communicating the status of the investigation

Issue: Care by a physician

Analysis: This letter does a good job of explaining the "peer review" process. It's succinct, but thorough and considerate, which is all it has to be.

[Date]

[Name]
[Address]

Dear ____________,

I wanted to follow-up with you regarding your concerns about your care by one of our physicians during your emergency department visit. We apologize for your experience and would like to inform you that every complaint is investigated thoroughly. At this point, I have completed my review of your complaint and have asked a physician to review the care you received. This peer review is currently underway and includes a review of the medical record and discussion with the physician involved. The peer review weighs your care against our expectations of the professional care received by our patients. I will contact you as soon as I learn the outcome of the peer review. I appreciate your patience.

Thank you again for bringing your concerns to our attention. If you have any questions please feel free to contact our department at [telephone number].

Sincerely,

[Name]
[Title]

Issue: Dispute about physician's treatment

Analysis: This letter reads "too official" and it is written without much consideration for the recipient's care. The opening paragraph should have been lower, as it tells the reader information they would expect. Also notice how the writer uses a passive tone in many of the sentences. For example, in the first sentence of the second paragraph, the writer says, "Mr. ____'s medical record was reviewed...." A better approach is to communicate what you've done through a more active style. Change this sentence to read like this: "We reviewed Mr. ____'s medical record as part of our quality and risk management protocol."

[Date]

[Name]
[Address]

Dear Mrs. ________,

[Name] Hospital is a health care facility that uses an integrated system of quality assurance, peer review and risk management. One of the goals is to monitor and improve the quality of the health care services we provide. Patient care is reviewed on an ongoing basis with established quality indicators that the nurse quality reviewers use.

Mr. [Name]'s medical record was reviewed as part of the quality and risk management protocol. The department staff, based on established criteria, reviewed his case. Based on the established criteria for review, they recommended that the medical record be submitted to the physician peer review process. This letter is to inform you that the care rendered and the events during his care is still being reviewed by the physician peer review process.

If you have any questions concerning the care that your husband received during his admission to [name of hospital] please contact me at [telephone number].

Sincerely,

[Name]
[Title]

Cc: [Name]

Issue: Poor outcome of obstetric case

Analysis: This letter's strong suit is how it details the review process and where this complaint stands within that process. However, despite the fact that the letter admits the complaint is still being reviewed, it pronounces this judgment, "While your difficulties are not something we would expect following any delivery, the committee does not see them as a result of any major error in diagnosis, judgment, technique or management." Be very careful and consider not including a final decision while a complaint is still in the process. Also, be careful when including a long list of people who received copies of this letter. Consider BCCing or providing a status memo to necessary recipients instead.

[Date]

[Name]
[Address]

Dear ___________,

I am writing this letter in response to your concerns relating to the care provided by Dr. [name of physician] to you in our emergency department on [date].

The clinical chief for obstetrics and the quality assurance/utilization committee of the medical staff are reviewing your concerns. They have completed the first part of the investigation (your medical care). It is certainly regretful that you have had to experience your degree of pain and the inconvenience of repeated visits to physicians since your delivery on [date]. While your difficulties are not something we would expect following any delivery, the committee does not see them as a result of any major error in diagnosis, judgment, technique or management.

Currently, the committee is discussing your case with Dr. [name of physician] and [name of physician]. It is important for physicians to conduct patient questioning in an empathetic and sensitive manner. The committee will evaluate how these physicians communicated with you and how we can improve that communication in the future. We will contact you with the outcome of that review.

It is our sincere desire to make all client contacts with programs and services offered by [name of organization] a positive experience. We appreciate the time you took to bring forward your concerns and are hopeful that any future contacts will be more positive.

Should you wish to discuss any of these matters further, please do not hesitate to contact me at [telephone number].

Yours sincerely,
[Name]
Director of Quality Care

c.c. Chief of Staff
Clinical Chief Obstetrics
Emergency Room Physician
Obstetrician
Family Physician
Regional Health Centre Coordinators
President/CEO

Issue: Iatrogenic injury discovered after discharge

Analysis: This letter takes the novel approach mentioned in Chapter 1, "Admitting liability? A novel approach." As mentioned in that chapter, this may reduce legal fees from lengthy litigation, result in a lower settlement, avoid punitive damages, prevent fraud allegations, improve its image in the community, etc. However, the key is determining whether it is appropriate at this time or in this case to use this approach. Because this complaint is still under review, it might be too early to admit liability. Ensure that this is the time and approach your hospital wishes to use.

[Date]

[Name]
[Address]

Dear____________,

Thank you for bringing your husband's experience at [facility name] to our attention. With the assistance of the quality management department, I have facilitated the review of this case by the chairman of the [physician section/department]. It is also under review by the [additional committee review, or chief of staff].

While [facility name] and other hospitals strive to provide the highest quality care, that is regrettably not always the case. In your husband's case, the most critical and life threatening injuries were treated without incident. Unfortunately, it does appear [description of iatrogenic injury or omission in care] was not discovered until after the more acute problems had been treated and your husband had been discharged.

I appreciate your concerns and thank you for bringing this matter to our attention. I also wish to apologize on behalf of our organization. We will contact you with the results of our investigation and an assurance of our performance improvement.

Sincerely,

[Name]
[Title]

Following-up with dissatisfied patients

Issue: Admitting and billing process

Analysis: This letter is in reply to a patient's calls with several staff at a hospital, and it has many strengths. The offer of waiving the second emergency bill is a good use of the discretionary fund here, as it appears the patient complained to several departments. The writer does a good job not admitting guilt, rather apologizing for the experience the patient had. The writer also mentions several ways the hospital will use the information from the complaint.

[Date]

[Name]
[Address]

Dear _____,

I am writing as a follow-up to your phone calls to me and to others in [Name of Department] regarding care you received in our emergency department. I understand that [Name of person] contacted you shortly after we spoke.

I have reviewed your concerns with the emergency department medical director and want to assure you that your concerns have been heard. Please accept my apology on behalf of [Name of Hospital]. As a gesture of good will, we will not bill you for the second visit to the emergency department. If you have already received a bill, please disregard it.

While we try very hard to provide excellent patient care every day, we do depend on our customers to identify areas for improvement. Please be assured that the medical director and emergency department management will follow up with staff on an individual basis.

I have also related your comments regarding the admitting and billing processes to the appropriate department managers for their review and action. They too will relate your observations regarding their respective processes to the individuals involved.

Although it may be of little consolation, I want to, again, apologize for any inconvenience this may have caused and to thank you for taking the time to contact us regarding this matter.

Sincerely,

[Name]
[Department]

Issue: Quality of care—response to patient call

Analysis: The apology came a bit late in this letter. Plus, there are too many "trust me, we'll address your concerns" type comments; people like to hear these, but when they're written several times in a letter, they suspect the comments are ingenuous. One positive: The writer gives very little detail here about the complaint, which may be good from a legal perspective. Also, though there's no hard and fast rule on carbon copying hospital staff on letters, some experts say a laundry list of staff under the "cc" line sends the wrong message to patients. It may look to patients as though the organization has simply tried to "cover all tracks."

[Date]

[Name]
[Address]

Dear ______,

Thank you for your contacting me regarding your concerns for the care provided by one of our staff members during your recent hospitalization. We appreciate you bringing these concerns to our attention, allowing us the opportunity to review our practice and respond.

Your expectation that each call be responded to promptly, courteously, and professionally is certainly reasonable, and indeed, our patients should expect nothing less. We expect all health care providers to treat patients with respect and consideration. We sincerely regret that this was not your experience. Although hospital personnel are afforded the same confidentiality as our patients, we want to assure you that the responsible administrative staff has taken appropriate follow up action with the employee.

We are grateful for patient feedback, as we recognize that problems that go unnoticed are missed opportunities for improvement. Our goal is to provide quality medical care with the warmth and compassion that our patients need and deserve. We are sorry for any additional strain this experience may have placed on you and appreciate the opportunity to look into this matter. If I can be of further assistance, please do not hesitate to contact me directly at [number and/or e-mail].

Sincerely,

[Name]
[Title]

cc: [Names and/or titles, e.g. LLL, Administrative Director, Critical Care & Med/Surg Services, SSS, Manager, Multi-Specialty Unit]

Issue: Quality of care—emergency room and radiology

Analysis: This letter does a good job of getting to the actions the hospital is taking to fix the problems, but it makes some mistakes in its explanations. First, patients don't necessarily know what's involved with "peer review" and what that process entails. "Overread" is another word that the writer should have clarified. The writer chose not to explain the results of peer review, which is appropriate to avoid legal issues, but probably should have shared the results about whether the timeline could be shortened.

Lastly, don't, as this writer did, follow the apology by "hoping" the patient will return; the patient will make that decision when and if the time comes. Instead, word this as "We want to be your family's health care system of choice. In the future we want to serve you and your family with the highest possible quality of care."

[Date]

[Name]
[Address]

Dear __________,

I am writing this letter as a follow-up to our telephone conversation and the contact made by your parents, [names]. Please accept my apology about the delay in my contacting you. Be assured that administration and the staff at [name] Hospital are concerned about providing a high level of quality care. Upon review of the concerns regarding your care in the emergency room I would like to outline the actions that I have taken, which are:

1. Physician peer review of the ER visit by the ER medical director.
2. Notification of the ER physician regarding the radiology over-read, its outcome and recommendations for improvement.
3. Review of the notification process to determine if the time line can be shortened.
4. Inform ER staff and social service of the referral availability of Dr. __________ regarding patients with Muscular Dystrophy;
5. Fax a copy of radiology report to Dr. ______________.
6. Send a copy of the x-ray to [name] Clinic to the attention of ____________.

I am truly sorry that you had such a negative experience and hope that you would give [name] Hospital a chance to provide quality service should you have a future need.

Thank you for your open discussion of your concerns. We always appreciate the opportunity to evaluate services, which have been provided to our customers and make appropriate improvements. Should you have any further questions please feel free to contact me at [telephone number].

Sincerely,

[Name]
[Title]

Issue: Suggestion for improvement in phlebotomy process

Analysis: This letter does an excellent job of congratulating the patient for their recommendations and expressing apology. This letter is in follow up to a phone conversation and it appears the writer has already explained the crux of the corrective actions taken here by the hospital's IV therapy unit.

[Date]

[Name]
[Address]

Dear ____________,

Thank you for giving me your feedback about your experience at [name of hospital]. As we have discussed, I sincerely regret our service did not exceed your expectations. Your opinion and comments are very important to us. In an effort to correct and improve our service, I have shared your concerns with the nurse involved and discussed specific ways that we could have better met your needs. I will continue to directly observe the unit to assure that corrections have been taken.

The IV therapy department staff is committed to continual improvement of our services and thank you again for taking the time to express your concerns. You have been helpful in assisting us to improve our overall care.

I hope you are doing well and are satisfied with the corrective measures we have taken. Should you have further concerns please contact me, [name], at [telephone number].

[Name] Health System wants to be your health care system of choice. In the future we look forward to continuing to serve you and your family with the highest possible quality of care.

Sincerely,

[Name]
[Title]

Issue: Quality and timeliness of care

Analysis: No specific details here, which weaken this letter. That said, the immediate introduction is helpful to give the reader some context. The title tells the patient that there is someone at the hospital who, like them, cares about improving performance. Details about the education are useful, as well, though the third paragraph should have been higher up. The second paragraph does not address the patient's concern directly; it would have been better in the closing.

[Date]

[Name]
[Address]

Dear Mr. ____________,

I am the director of performance improvement for [name] Hospital. I received your letter of [date] detailing your concerns about your care. I thank you for offering your recollections and criticisms of your care and I am grateful that you have taken the time and effort to inform us of your experience. I believe your comments are valid and deserve a response.

Service quality is extremely important at [name] Hospital and we are happy that you gave us the opportunity to follow up on your experience. While it is disappointing that you were dissatisfied with several aspects of your care, such letters are very important to us because they offer an opportunity to see how others view us. Ultimately, we hope that each and every letter of complaint may lead to improvement in the care we render at [name] Hospital.

There is no doubt that you suffered through a very trying and difficult time during your hospitalization. The experience had to have been most stressful, beyond what can be expressed in words. Let me assure you that we believe all patients, families and visitors should be treated with respect and dignity and that each patient is afforded the highest level of care possible. In the past few months, several new programs have been instituted that will have a positive effect on the quality and timeliness of the care provided to our patients and their families. These programs are grounded in ethics, excellence in care collaboration, and respect. They reinforce to our employees the need to be courteous, reliable and professional while adhering to the high standards our institution has historically set forth. Patient satisfaction is very important to [name] Hospital and to the staff. Through staff meetings, in-services and staff supervision, we are working with the staff to heighten their awareness of how patient care is perceived and to be more sensitive and responsive to patients' needs.

Once again, we thank your for your letter. We are sorry we did not meet your expectation. It is through letters such as yours, that we are able to identify areas for review of our processes and hopefully improve upon them.

Sincerely,

[Name]
[Title]

Issue: Testing, diagnosis and quality of care

Analysis: Letter describes in excellent detail each patient concern and provides in basic terms an explanation for each. The writer could have done more to explain "why" the billed charges could not be removed.

[Date]

[Name]
[Address]

Dear _______________,

Thank you for taking the time to contact us about your mother's, [patient name], recent visit to [name] Hospital. We were sorry to learn that our services did not meet your expectations. We appreciate the information you have shared with us so that we may continue to improve our services.

Our medical director has reviewed [patient name] medical record in detail and the diagnosis of both pneumonia and congestive heart failure were identified and treated within accepted clinical parameters. Both radiology and laboratory testing confirmed these diagnoses. As you know, the patient's dementia complicated her ability to provide history of pain or discomfort or to participate fully in her care. We acknowledge your concerns regarding the inconsistent communications within the hospital. We are working with our employees and physicians to improve the consistency of communications with patients and families.

The concerns about fluids, pain management and restraints were also reviewed. The chart review revealed that a variety of medications were administered to manage the symptoms you mention. Restraints are applied in circumstances where the risk of injury or harm is significant. They are carefully monitored and removed as quickly as the situation allows.

I have shared your concerns with the individuals who were involved with [patient name] care in detail. The emergency department's quality team has reviewed both your concerns regarding the emergency department and the billed charges received. It has been determined that the charges are accurate as the tests were performed. Therefore, the billed charges will not be reduced.

We thank you again for taking the time to share your concerns and apologize that we did not meet your expectations. If you should need assistance during any future encounters, please feel free to ask to speak to the house supervisor or contact administration.

Sincerely,

[Name]
[Title]

Responding to patients when family members complain

Issue: Patient's mother passed along complaint about hospital's handout and care

Analysis: Excellent letter because the writer tells the complainant exactly what the OB unit has done with her suggestion and why. It admits to a problem with communication and moves on, focusing on the efforts underway to improve the booklet.

[Date]

[Name]
[Address]

Dear ______________,

I am writing to follow up about the concerns your mother, [name], communicated to us regarding your [date] admission to the [name] Hospital.

All staff involved, as well as members of the district management team, have reviewed the concerns. We recognize patients present themselves to us in vulnerable situations and need to be assured that their needs will be looked after. As a result of our review, we see opportunity for us to improve both what and how we are communicating with patients.

The handout you were provided has been discontinued. Members of our obstetrical team—including public health nurses and a consumer advocate—are currently working on a booklet that will have a client-centered approach and provide useful information to clients using the obstetrical services.

Our apologies to you for the unpleasant experiences you faced during your care here. It is our sincere desire to ensure that all clients positively experience the programs and services offered by the [name] Hospital. We appreciate the time your mother took to bring forward your concerns and are hopeful that as a result of our review, future contacts will be more positive for yourself and/or others receiving our services.

Should you wish to discuss any of these matters further, please do not hesitate to contact me at [phone number].

Sincerely,

[Name]
[Title]

Issue: Family member complained about lack of communication from staff

Analysis: Lots of praise in this letter, which is good; the early apology is also effective. The final paragraph is a much better way to tell the family member that you want them to come back, compared with the line in the earlier letter ("We hope you give us a chance.")

[Date]

[Name]
[Address]

Dear Mr. ___________________,

Thank you for sharing information about your recent experience when you brought your mother, [name], to [name] Hospital. We sincerely regret our service did not meet your expectations. Your opinion is very important to us.

The care concerns we discussed on the phone are being addressed with the nursing staff involved in your mother's care. I will also have our medical director talk with the emergency department physician who cared for your mother. Staff has been reminded of the expected communication that should occur with patients and families regarding their treatment plans and the need for regular updates.

We are committed to continual improvement of our service and thank you again for taking the time to express your concerns. You have been helpful in assisting us to improve our performance.

We hope your mother is doing well and you are satisfied with the corrective measures we have taken. Should you have further concerns please contact me, [name] at [telephone number].

We want to be your family's health care system of choice. In the future we want to serve you and your family with the highest possible quality of care.

Sincerely,

[Name]
[Title]

CHAPTER 8

Closure Replies: Responding with the Final Decision and Results of the Investigation

CHAPTER 8

Closure Replies: Responding with the Final Decision and Results of the Investigation

This chapter contains sample letters for one of the most important steps in the process to resolve patient complaints: communicating the results of an investigation and providing closure for the situation. Resolving complaints means good customer service and in turn, good business. Angela Burnette, an attorney and author of Chapter 1 says, "How a hospital addresses a patient's complaint undoubtedly affects the chances a patient will later file a lawsuit against the hospital or report the problem to a government agency." Consider the sample letters in this chapter and our analysis of them.

Follow-up letters responding to a complaint with apologies, actions taken, and corrective measures

Analysis: The letters in this section do an excellent job of communicating resolution, particularly in cases in which the outcome is not one the patient wants. In these more delicate letters, it's best to recap the process you took as an institution—and you personally—to reach the resolution. Discuss in some detail the actions you took or plan to take and corrective measures. Do not simply say that you are fixing the problem; the complainant deserves to know how. Pay close attention to the letter, "Issue: Apologies and corrective measure," in this section.

Issue: Uncomfortable phlebotomy procedure—corrective measures taken

Background: Sample letter sent directly to the patient who complained regarding the phlebotomy process and not having a pillow or board placed as a comfort measure under their arm during the process.

[Date]

[Name]
[Address]

RE: [Subject line and/or case number]

Dear ___________,

Thank you for giving me your feedback about your experience at [Name of hospital]. As we have discussed, I sincerely regret our service did not exceed your expectations. Your opinion and comments are very important to us. In an effort to correct and improve our service, I have shared your concerns with the nurse involved and discussed specific ways that we could have better met your needs. I will continue to directly observe the unit to assure that corrections have been taken.

The IV Therapy Department staff is committed to continual improvement of our services and thank you again for taking the time to express your concerns. You have been helpful in assisting us to improve our overall care.

I hope you are doing well and are satisfied with the corrective measures we have taken. Should you have further concerns please contact me, [name], at [phone number] or [name], Chief Operating Officer at [phone number].

[Hospital name] wants to be your health care system of choice. In the future we look forward to continuing to serve you and your family with the highest possible quality of care.

Sincerely,

[Name]
[Title]
[Department]

Issue: Location and waiting area—apologies and corrective measures

[Date]

[Name]
[Address]

RE: [Subject line and/or case number]

Dear _________,

Thank you for sharing your MRI experience with me last week. I understand the anxiety and fear that can accompany any kind of health care event and I apologize that you had such a difficult encounter.

As promised, I am writing to let you know of the resolution to the problems you encountered. First, in regards to finding your way around the campus, I recognize that our campus is difficult at best to navigate. As I mentioned to you, a subcommittee has been convened to address this issue. Some of the initiatives that are being proposed to improve patients' and family members' way-finding experiences include:

- Providing maps at integral locations throughout the facility
- Arming our staff with maps and improved training regarding locating different departments
- Asking all departments to provide walking directions for patients from the various streets and parking garages surrounding [Hospital name]
- Improving signage throughout the facility
- Posting greeters at different entrances to help provide patients with directions to their destinations.

Second, I contacted [Name], Director of Outpatient Radiology. She indicated that there is a second overflow waiting area in the rear of the radiology department where patients should have been directed. She was concerned that patients were forced to sit on the floor and is informing her staff to direct patients to the overflow area when necessary. She also provided her staff with feedback regarding appropriate discussion in front of patients. She informed staff that arguments regarding a patient's clinical treatment should never be discussed in front of a patient.

I hope that these actions will ensure that all of our patients continue to receive high quality and caring treatment from [Hospital name]. If you have any further questions or concerns, please don't hesitate to contact me directly at [phone number].

Best Regards,

[Name]
[Title]

Issue: Poor care—apologies and gift certificate offered

[Date]

[Name]
[Address]

RE: [Subject line and/or case number]

Dear __________,

Thank you for contacting us with your concerns relating to services that you received from [Clinic name]. Your complete satisfaction is very important to us. We appreciate your comments. Your input gives us the opportunity to review our services and make changes where necessary. You contacted us about [describe the situation].

We regret that you had this experience and we have followed up on your comments and have thoroughly discussed the situation with the appropriate personnel.

Please accept my apologies for your inconvenience. I have included a gift certificate for your use on behalf of [Clinic name]. This in no way can justify the dissatisfaction that you described from your visit at our facility. It is our commitment to do everything possible to ensure that this situation does not occur in the future.

Thank you again for taking the time to share your concerns. If I can be of assistance in the future, please call me at [phone number].

Sincerely,

[Name]
[Title]

Issue: Delayed mammography results—corrective actions taken

[Date]

[Name]
[Address]

RE: [Subject line and/or case number]

Dear ___________,

Thank you for sharing your [Hospital name] mammography experience with me today. I understand the anxiety and fear that can accompany the waiting for results of a mammogram and I apologize that you had such a difficult experience.

As promised, I am writing to let you know of the resolution to the problems you encountered. I spoke with [Name], Director of Outpatient Radiology, who oversees [Hospital name] radiology services. She is taking the following actions to ensure that our patients receive the appropriate care each and every time they visit [Hospital name].

1. Mammography technologists will communicate to patients that a radiologist must review the mammogram film before the final results are released to the patient. The results will be sent to the patient by mail. It is a legal requirement that results are reported by written communication to protect patient confidentiality.

2. The process by which letters are sent to patients communicating the outcome of their mammograms is being reviewed to ensure that each patient receives the appropriate communication.

3. The process by which patients are sent reminders to make appointments for routine mammograms is being reviewed and revised.

Additionally, I wanted to inform you that there is a radiologist on duty most of the time at our [Hospital name] radiology center. However, the radiologist is not always able to meet personally with each patient.

I hope that these actions will ensure that all of our patients continue to receive high quality and caring treatment from our [Hospital name] facility. If you have any further questions or concerns, please don't hesitate to contact me directly at [phone number].

Regards,

[Name]
[Title]

Issue: Mammogram reminder notice sent to mastectomy patient—apologies

[Date]

[Name]
[Address]

RE: [Subject line and/or case number]

Dear __________,

This is a follow up to the issue you brought to my attention in the Complaints Department at [Hospital name] on [date].

The issue was regarding a mammogram reminder notice that you recently received. You stated that there should be a system in place for members who have had a double mastectomy not to receive this type of reminder.

Through my investigation I discovered that [Hospital name] is currently instituting ways of identifying members who have had a double mastectomy. This program has not yet been fully implemented.

In the meantime, I have taken the appropriate steps to have your name manually removed from the list of members receiving mammogram reminders. It is understandable how emotionally upsetting this reminder was for you considering your situation.

Thank you for taking the time to bring this issue to our attention, [Hospital name] would like to apologize for this unfortunate reminder. If you would like to contact me to discuss this further you can reach me directly at [telephone number]. If you prefer, my e-mail address is: [e-mail address]

Sincerely,

[Name]
[Title]

Issue: Pediatric transfer—apologies and follow-up

[Date]

[Name]
[Address]

RE: [Subject line and/or case number]

Dear ___________,

Thank you for making us aware of the situation that occurred on [date] with the pediatric transfer of your son [name] from our hospital. We strive to provide high quality patient care, when we are not successful in this endeavor we want to know about it so that we can review the situation and make appropriate improvements where indicated.

We have reviewed your son's records and discussed this situation with [Doctor's name]. Unfortunately, it appears that there was a breakdown in communication between [Doctor' name] and our hospital ER physician. We will be monitoring this department's physician on-call process and communications for opportunities for improvement and to reduce the likelihood of a reoccurrence.

We apologize for this situation and any inconvenience or aggravation that it has caused. We are glad that the appropriate referral was made to [Doctor's name], that your son was admitted at another hospital, and is now doing much better. We hope that you will continue to have [patient's name] seen by [Doctor's name] or [Doctor's name].

Again, thank you for making us aware of the situation and your concerns. We will monitor the process to assure high quality of care in the future. Please let me know if we can be of further assistance.

Sincerely,

[Name]
[Title]

Results of investigations

Analysis: Writing these letters can be tricky, as they are filled with legal risks. Often, the patient is right, and when there is guilt for the everyday types of mistakes that can happen, you must find a way to apologize, but not admit culpability. The third letter in this section about a patient's fall does a good job of this.

Issue: Patients claimed rights were violated (two letters)

Letter 1: Room assignments

[Date]

[Name]
[Address]

RE: [Complaint #]

Dear ____________,

Thank you for bringing this concern to our attention. This letter will explain the outcome of our investigation. In addition, we will be responding to the complainant via letter.

[Patient name] registered this complaint on her own behalf as a patient of the specific Unit at [Hospital name]. The complaint was that she stated her rights were being violated.

As evidenced in our documentation, on [date] [patient name] first asked to be moved to the new directions unit and was told that there were no beds available. On [date] she called, leaving a phone message about moving, stating that her [specify patient right] was being violated. (See the patient bill of rights enclosed). During the follow up phone call to the message, she stated that she had discovered that a private room on [room location] was being cleaned following a patient discharge and wanted to have the room.

It was then explained to [patient name] that the room had been assigned the day before to a new admission so there was still no room available and that she would need an order from her physician to be moved. She also was reminded that rooms were assigned based on patient needs. She demanded to know what those needs were and it was explained that due to confidentiality her wish could not be granted. [Patient name] then became angry and told the patient advocate to leave her room and not return. She stated that in her opinion, the patient advocate was not good and she was going to report her, and added that she had requested the room yesterday prior to anyone else.

The charge nurse said that she began asking on the morning of [date] and that the assignment had been made the night before pending discharge of the current resident. She said that she tried to explain to [patient name] that there is no seniority list and that beds are assigned according to need. In addition, beds are assigned by need first and request when possible. Following this discussion, [patient name] told the nurse to leave. The nurse left as requested, and thus the conversation ended.

[Doctor name], the Medical Director performed his review of the situation and rendered the following opinions:

- He was familiar with this patient and had observed her behavior on a number of occasions.
- He found the actions taken to be appropriate.
- He also recommended that the Psychiatric Joint Practice Committee review the process for dealing with difficult acting-out patients.

During the investigative process it was determined that the patient to whom the room was assigned had a more urgent need for a private room. As per policy, the room assignment was made based on the needs of the new patient.

I hope this serves to clarify any questions regarding this complaint.

Sincerely,

[Name], [Credentials]
[Department]
[Hospital]

Letter 2: Private room assignment

[Date]

[Name]
[Address]

RE: [Subject line and/or case number]

Dear _______________,

This is in regard to your concern over your rights while being a patient at [Hospital name] unit on [dates].

First of all, we would like to extend our gratitude to you for bringing your concern to our attention. We want to assure you that we did a thorough investigation and that we do our absolute best to provide accommodations that our clients will find pleasant, safe and supportive during their stay.

The results of our investigation showed that most of our rooms are semi-private and that we cannot always honor requests for private rooms when someone with more acute needs is admitted. The safety and immediate needs of the client are foremost in room assignments and we are obligated by confidentiality to not reveal personal details in order to explain those needs.

In addition, your physician approved of your room assignment taking your best health interest into consideration. Furthermore, the medical director has also performed a review of the concern and has concluded that he concurs with the decision that was made.

I hope this answers your concerns and we look forward to providing care to you and your family in the future should the need arise.

Sincerely,

[Name], [Credentials]
[Title]
[Hospital]

Issue: Patient fell

[Date]

[Name]
[Address]

RE: [Subject line and/or case number]

Dear ________________,

This is in regard to your concern about the care that [name] received while she was a patient on the [Hospital name] on [dates].

First of all, we would like to extend our gratitude to you for bringing your concern to our attention. We want to assure you that we did a thorough investigation and that we do our absolute best to provide care and accommodations that our clients will find pleasant, safe and supportive during their stay.

The results of our investigation are as follows:

- The facility is cleaned on a regular basis and due to the nature of the illness of our patient's there are sometimes accidents o the floor/beds etc. The environmental services department keeps a comprehensive log of the cleaning tasks that are performed on a regular basis and in addition keep track of the calls that come in reporting these instances. Their response time averages 30 minutes.
- A review of the medical record revealed that she did fall and that she was fully clothed with dress shoes on and was attempting to pick up wet towels. She did sustain a laceration, which was cleaned, and then she was transferred to the emergency department where the laceration was stitched and she was evaluated for any other injuries as well as for the cause of the fall.
- She had not received any medication prior to the fall that would have rendered her unable to maintain her balance.
- Her physician performed an examination and documented that she was responding to her current therapy regimen.
- As for long-term care, the [Hospital name] is not a long-term placement facility and when any patient reaches certain criteria they must be discharged. The criteria are set by a regulatory agency.

I hope this answers your concerns and we look forward to providing care to you and your family in the future should the need arise.

Sincerely,

[Name], [Credentials]
[Title]
[Hospital]

Issue: Attitude of and care by medical staff issue

[Date]

[Name of Recipient]
[Street address]
[City, State Zip code]

RE:[Subject line and/or case number]

Dear [Name]:

I am writing today in response to concerns about your hospitalization from [dates] that your son, [name of concerned party], brought to both my attention and that of [name], our chief executive officer. After speaking with [name of concerned party], I forwarded his concerns to [name], nurse manager of [department name], and to [doctor name] of the emergency department. Listed below are [patient's name] concerns along with the responses that I received.

- [Doctor's name] did not seem confident: [doctor's name] recalled seeing you and in his opinion, he felt that you could be reevaluated for your condition in 24 hours after receiving treatment on the first visit. [Doctor's name] informed you of the hours he would be in the emergency department the following day and you did in fact present to the emergency department the next day where [doctor's name] reexamined you. When [doctor's name] used the word deliberate he was referring to the fact that he would have to find an attending physician to admit you as he had no intention of discharging you after seeing you again on Sunday. [Doctor's name] will, in the future, try to explain himself more clearly when he is communicating with patients and their families.

- General attitude of the staff [hospital department]: Treating our patients and their families with respect should be one of our top priorities. Apparently in this particular instance we failed on our part to show a caring and respectful attitude. This will not be tolerated, and according to [name], nurse manager, she says, "Anyone displaying these types of behaviors will be counseled and discipline initiated."

- Medication and orders consistently late/long wait before call was answered: [Name], nurse manager is currently reviewing both of these issues. When medication and orders are not given according to policy, the specific reason will be documented and explained to the patient and family members.

- [Patient name] was yelled at for taking her own medication: The nursing staff should have explained why you could not take your own medication. Your physician would actually need to write an order allowing you to take your own medication, and the pharmacy department would need to check any medication brought in by patients or their families. I apologize that you were yelled at. We should have taken the time to communicate with you and explain [name] Hospital's position on allowing patients to take their own medication.

I was made aware that [name], nurse manager spoke with you prior to your being discharged about many of the concerns [concerned party name] brought to our attention. Hopefully you found that conversation to be worthwhile and [name of nurse manager] was able to answer any questions you may have had. Please know that [name of nurse manager] has shared all of [name of concerned party] concerns with her staff during recent staff meetings and will be monitoring the staff on an ongoing basis.

On behalf of [CEO name], [doctor's name], [name of nurse manager] and myself, I wish to thank you and [Name of concerned party] for sharing your concerns with us. Although we cannot go back and change the incidents that occurred while you were at our facility, hopefully we can make a difference for our future patients.

If I can be of further assistance to you or [name of concerned party], please feel free to contact me at [telephone number].

Sincerely,

[Name]
[Title]

Cc: [Names of all involved people]

Issue: Standard of care—hospital found it was met

[Date]

[Name]
[Address]

RE: [Subject line and/or case number]

Dear ______________,

As director of quality management, your letter to [name] dated [date], was given to me for review. Be assured that administration and the staff at [hospital name] are concerned about providing a high level of quality care. Upon review of the concerns outlined in your letter I have thoroughly examined your medical record and determined that the care provided in the emergency department was appropriate and the appropriate standard of care was met. The physician, who is not an employee of the hospital that provided your care, is fully qualified and credentialed. As a result of this evaluation of your care and treatment there will be no change in the bill for services provided. There also is no reason to sanction the physician who provided your care.

I am sorry that you experienced the pain that you described. Infections in wounds of this type are not uncommon and the physician that provided your care prescribed appropriate medications regarding this concern. Upon discharge from the emergency department you were appropriately instructed regarding the potential for infection and advised to report back to the emergency department or your personal physician if you experience any symptoms of infection.

Thank you for your letter. We always appreciate the opportunity to evaluate services, which have been provided to our customers and make appropriate improvements. Should you have any further questions please feel free to contact me at [telephone number].

Sincerely,

[Name]
[Title]

CC: [Recipient of original]

Issue: Inability to review medical records

[Date]

[Name]
[Address]

RE: [Subject line and/or case number]

Dear ________________,

Thank you for taking the time to tell us about your concerns with our response to your request to review your wife's medical records during her stay at our facility. Our grievance committee has reviewed your concerns and conducted a full investigation into the issues.

After investigating your concerns, it was determined that our response to your request was appropriate and followed our policy guidelines. Although we determined that our response was appropriate, we do realize that we did not meet your expectations.

The hospital will review the procedure for responding to requests to review medical records after usual business hours in an attempt to better serve our customers.

Our mission is one of a compassionate and healing environment for all patients. It is most disappointing that your perception was otherwise. The hospital certainly appreciates the opportunity to address the concerns you have brought to our attention.

If I may be of service to you or your family, please contact me directly [phone number].

Sincerely,

[Name]
[Title]
[Department]

Issue: Quality of food in long-term care facility

[Date]

[Name]
[Address]

RE: [Subject line and/or case study]

Dear ________________,

I am writing in follow-up to our discussions on [date]. Thank you for taking the time to share your concerns related to the quality of food and care at [name of organization]. Feedback from residents and their families is important as the organization strives to provide the best care and service possible.

I have been unsuccessful in contacting you at your home phone number and have been reluctant to interrupt you at work by calling you on your cell phone. Therefore, I am communicating by letter and trust that if you have any further questions, comments or concerns that you will call me to either further discuss on the phone or set-up an appointment.

I have investigated your concerns with staff at name of organization and would like to share with you the following:

- **Bacon**
  It is unfortunate your mother was served bacon that was undercooked and our apologies for that. At the name of organization, bacon is cooked in a convection oven, which is the best way to distribute the heat evenly. As well, staff follow standard cooking times, etc., to ensure proper food preparation. As you had noted you had viewed a pan that was "nicely done" and feedback from others that day has also suggested the bacon was "nicely done". It would seem that the undercooked bacon was an exception to the majority of the bacon that was served on that day. However, the discussion around the concern has been helpful and staff will continue to monitor to minimize the likelihood of any future occurrence. We also recognize that sometimes one resident may like bacon more cooked than others, and staff try to accommodate such requests. On every occasion, residents have the choice of a substitute item as well.

  While reviewing this concern area, we noted that you had some concerns about your mother's chewing and the fitting of her dentures. With this in mind, the food services manager has suggested that your mother be further assessed by the occupational therapist at name of organization.

- **Soup temperature**
  The setting out of soup at the tables prior to the residents sitting down at the tables is done as a safety precaution. Many residents are a bit shaky and many have reduced sensation and could easily burn themselves if they don't recognize how hot something is. Staff take the temperature of the soup after it is cooked and while it is holding in the steam table to ensure the right soup temperature. We also have taken the soup temperature at the resident tables over a three-day period and temperatures have ranged from 160-165 degrees, which is within acceptable standards.

- **Undercooked and overcooked vegetables, etc.**
  Staff have acknowledged that this has been a problem area in the past and a new steamer has recently been purchased which should minimize such occurrences in the future. Also, standardized recipes are in place for all foods to ensure consistency in food preparation at the nursing home.

- **Waste of food**
  There is ongoing monitoring of plate returns and changes are made to the menu accordingly. There is usually a "second choice" if a resident does not like a particular item being served. To ensure adequate nutrition, resident weights are monitored every three months and more frequently if a problem is identified.

- **Quality of food**
  Staff have very strict specifications regarding the quality of food that is acceptable for ordering to ensure standards are maintained. As we discussed, if there is a particular item of concern, please do not hesitate to bring it forward to [name], Food Services Manager at [telephone number].

For many of the residents, food services staff recognize that meal time is the highlight of the day, so they understand how important it is to listen and try to accommodate resident wishes. The food services manager attends meetings at least twice a year to gain direct resident/family feedback. Many of the concern areas you have brought forward were identified at the last meeting and further discussion of these concern areas will take place with the food services manager at the next staff and resident meeting. You are encouraged to directly contact the food services manager on any concerns related to nutrition and quality of food service.

Other general care issues have been brought to the attention of staff (e.g., resident bedtimes, respect being shown to residents, minimal evening activity programming, etc.). It is expected that all interactions between staff, residents and families be carried out in a respectful manner.

Staff have also received feedback from residents and/or families that they want to go to bed earlier and in many instances staff have found it challenging to encourage residents to stay up for the evening programming that does occur. The scenario you described of a resident requesting to watch TV and being refused should not be happening. The nursing unit manager would appreciate hearing the details should you have any further observations.

At the next staff and resident meeting, we will seek further feedback from residents/families on the activity program. The name of organization will continue to make every effort to accommodate resident preferences.

The review and discussion of all your concerns has been beneficial. As we discussed, it is important for the manager to know of concerns as close to the time of occurrence as possible. When the manager is not there, families are encouraged to discuss their concerns with the nurse in charge and/or leave a message for the manager to call them.

It is our sincere desire to make all client contacts with programs and services offered by the name of organization a positive experience. Concerns are an opportunity for us to review and improve the way we deliver services and once again we certainly appreciate the time you took to outline your concerns. I hope that our review meets with your satisfaction.

If you should have any further questions or concerns, please do not hesitate to contact me at [phone number].

Yours sincerely,

[Name]
[Title]

cc: [All involved parties]

Issue: Patient transfer

[Date]

[Name]
[Address]

RE: [Subject line and/or case study]

Dear_______________,

I am contacting you regarding your concern about the transfer of [patient name] to [hospital name] terminating his [date] admission to [name of unit] at [hospital name].

We would like to thank you for bringing this concern to our attention. It is our intention to provide the highest quality care possible. We performed an investigation upon receipt of your concern and the following are the results of that investigation:

- According to the medical record, [patient name] was deemed competent. Therefore, he was able to make a decision regarding the transfer independently.
- There is no medical record documentation entry with regard to the patient's permission to involve the family in his care planning or discharge process.
- [Patient name] had had no medication prior to discharge that would have impaired his decision making ability.
- It is standard of practice that [department name] benefited patients are sent to [name of unit]
- We have begun to look at our process for documentation and for obtaining patients permission to involve their families and or caregivers in their care planning and discharge processes.

It is our hope that this answers your concerns and we look forward to providing care to your family should the need arise.

Sincerely,

[Name]
[Title]

Letters pertaining to billing resolutions

Issue: Multiple insurance companies and collection suit

[Date]

[Name]
[Address]

RE: [Subject line and/or case number]

Dear_______________,

You contacted us on [date] to express your concern about our billing practices, specifically with regard to [name of patient] who was a patient in our emergency department at [name of hospital] on [date], following a motor vehicle accident.

This letter serves as notice of the results of our investigation into this matter.

First of all, we would like to extend our gratitude to you for bringing your concern to our attention. We want to assure you that we did a thorough investigation and that we do our absolute best to provide accommodations and practices that our clients will find efficient, safe and supportive.

The following is the result of our investigation:

We billed the visit to the patient's group insurance following the ER visit. We then found out from the patient's stepmother that we needed to bill [Name of automobile insurance] since this was a motor vehicle accident. We submitted a claim for the visit and received payment for a portion of the bill. We then rebilled the patient's group plan for the remainder of the bill. The group paid a portion, which left the patient with a balance that he was obligated to pay [State per what terms and how those had been shared with the patient].

The bill was then combined at collections with another account that this same patient owed. After several messages were left to try to find out why the payments had not been made, the collection agent filed suit. Following this, the patient began to make payments began and has continued to pay regularly.

We apologize for any confusion or delay that this process caused you and your family and sincerely hope that it has been resolved to your satisfaction. We look forward to providing care to you and your family in the future should the need arise.

Sincerely,

[Name]
[Title]
[Hospital name]

Issue: Billing error for service not received

[Date]

[Name]
[Address]

RE: [Subject line and/or case number]

Dear ____________,

I have tried reaching you via phone without success regarding the concerns you had about your emergency care center visit of [date].

I want you to be aware that follow-up pertaining to your billing question about [specify service] has been completed. Findings were that you did not receive this service. I have followed up with the patient accounting department to be sure your bill has been corrected regarding this matter. Your responsibility once this correction has been made will be your co-payment.

If you would like a copy of your medical record for this visit, you will need to contact our medical information services at [telephone number]. They will be able to help you with this matter.

I want to thank you for sharing your concerns. It is through this process that we can review and improve our services. I hope this follow-up has been helpful. Please feel free to call me at [telephone number] with any questions.

Sincerely,

[Name]
[Title]

Issue: Contesting tests and bills for tests

[Date]

[Name]
[Address]

RE: [Subject line and/or case number]

Dear ________________,

Your complaint was referred to me by [Name], director of patient care services. Based on the information contained within the file it appears that you presented to our emergency department on [date] with complaints of severe chest pain radiating up to your left shoulder. You were seen and treated by [doctor's name], who determined that your pain was not cardiac in nature. She ordered a chest x-ray, which revealed findings consistent with left lower lobe atelectasis, possibly a pulmonary embolism. At that point, a ventilation perfusion scan was ordered, which came back "indeterminate".

She contacted [doctor 2's name], who assumed responsibility for your care and admitted you to the hospital, because your symptoms continued to persist despite treatment with various medications in the emergency room. [Doctor 2's name] continued to order diagnostic studies in order to rule out pulmonary embolism. He ordered an ultrasound scan of your legs to rule out deep vein thrombosis, and later a pulmonary angiogram to obtain a definitive diagnosis.

Once he ruled out a lung embolism, he determined that the cause of your pain was due to a left lower lobe pneumonia, and he continued to treat you with antibiotics. Your record indicates that you did continue to complain of chest pain, and also experienced some right upper quadrant pain. Dr. [name] wanted to rule out a possible problem with your gallbladder and liver, and ordered an ultrasound. This subsequently came back negative and you were discharged on [date].

[Name] indicated that you are contesting your bill and the treatment and tests that were ordered by your physician. After thorough review, I believe that you were billed appropriately for services rendered. It is also my belief that the treatment prescribed by [doctor's name] was appropriate, given the clinical symptoms that you presented with in the emergency room and the diagnostic results that [doctor 2's name] was presented with throughout your hospital course.

Based on the available information, I must decline your demand that we rescind our charges. Our charges were for services that we provided in good faith and in accordance with community standards.

Should you have any further concerns or comments, please feel free to contact me at [telephone number].

Sincerely,

[Name]
[Title]

Issue: Complaint about poor care results in refund

[Date]

[Name]
[Address]

RE: Patient Complaint

Dear ________________,

Thank you for taking the time to meet with [doctor's name] and me to discuss your concerns regarding care received at our facility. As we discussed, we take these opportunities to address situations within our facility where we could be performing better. You willingness to share your experience and your perspective will impact how we deal with similar situations in the future.

As indicated, I am enclosing a refund check in the amount of [dollar amount]. Although you did indicate that the money was a secondary issue, I agree that it is the fair and equitable thing to do. I apologize for any misunderstanding and hope that this will allow us to bring this issue to a close.

I again wish to express, on behalf of the staff and leadership of [hospital name], our sincere apologies for any inconvenience you may have experienced. I would further re-emphasize my sincere appreciation for your willingness to bring this to my attention.

Should you have any questions, please do not hesitate to contact me at [telephone number].

Sincerely,

[Name]
[Title]

Issue: Complaint about test results—bill rescinded as goodwill gesture

[Date]

[Name]
[Address]

RE: [Subject line and/or case study]

Dear ______________,

Thank you for your letter of [date] and bringing your concern to our attention. We want to be made aware when our patients are not happy with the quality of care that they have received, so that we can review the situation and hopefully improve patient care when indicated.

We have reviewed your concern and the records with [doctor's name] from name of radiology corporation and [doctor 2's name]. They stand by the interpretations of the testing that was done here and the care rendered. We believe your care was appropriate. You were scheduled for a follow-up angiogram on [date], but chose to cancel it and go to another hospital for a second opinion.

As a gesture of goodwill only we are writing off the remaining patient balance due on your account of [dollar amount].

Please let me know if I can be of further assistance to you, [telephone number]

Sincerely,

[Name]
[Title]

Section III

How to Respond to Complex Grievances

Section III Contents

Chapter 9

Replies: Addressing Medical Staff and Hospital Errors

CHAPTER 9

Replies: Addressing Medical Staff and Hospital Errors

Introduction

Please carefully read Chapter 1, "Responding to patient complaints: Legal requirements and issues," if you haven't already. This chapter will provide your best guidance to addressing hospital and medical staff errors in writing. For your convenience, we've included again in this chapter the tips from that chapter about admitting error.

Figure 9.1 Nine Crucial Tips: Issues to Think About When Considering Whether to Openly Admit Liability

1. Assess whether an "error" really happened and be sure. While the patient is still hospitalized, the hospital may believe (but may not actually know) what truly happened. Two weeks later, the hospital may discover the incident was not really an error, or discover that an error occurred but it was the fault of a person or entity other than the hospital.
2. Determine whether the "error" was actually the proximate cause of any harm. For example, a hospital could have made a mistake, but it did not cause any harm or was unrelated to the harm that occurred.
3. Evaluate whether everyone at the hospital is "on board" and "on the same page" with making an admission. This means the hospital, physicians, and staff involved in the incident/complaint all agree as to what happened, that an error occurred, and that an admission should be made. The hospital should not respond to a patient complaint by making an admission, if others involved in the patient's care are still disagreeing about what happened.
4. Assess the chance a lawsuit would be filed by the patient or family. Many hospitals handle such conversations under the assumption a lawsuit will be filed.
5. Identify the best person to deliver the news to the patient or family. (Sometimes, the treating physician may not be the best person to talk with the family, due to the physician's demeanor or, perhaps, his or her inability to accept and admit responsibility.)
6. Also, the hospital should consider adopting a written policy describing who can attend such a meeting between the hospital and the patient or family. For example, a hospital may want to consider having a chaplain present.
7. Before making an admission, the hospital should talk with its insurance company regarding any "cooperation" or anti-admission clauses in the hospital's insurance policy. These clauses may affect whether an insurance company later tries to deny coverage for an incident.
8. If the decision has been made to admit an error, consider communicating such admissions out of benevolence/sympathy or as an attempt to negotiate a settlement or compromise of the dispute (discussed below) in order to help protect such statements from later being admitted as evidence.
9. If the decision has been made to admit an error, take care not to waive or disclose peer review privileged information (or attorney-client privileged information).

Responding to a case: Incident but no error

Issue: Grievance regarding care of daughter and facilities

Analysis: This letter provides quite a bit of detail about investigative results. Before sending out a letter like this, ensure that it "passes muster" with your hospital's legal requirements; you don't want to admit culpability in a letter. Your hospital might prefer disclosing findings in a more general way. This letter also is slightly condescending and brusque in its explanations, for example, "This issue is not due to an outdated saw but rather due to a lack of padding on the initial cast (applied at [name of other hospital])." Softer wording such as, "I can understand your concern that the wound was caused by an outdated saw. However, I want to reassure you that our saws are [checked per regulation]..." might be best. However, the letter's strength is its opening and closing.

[Date]

[Name]
[Address]

Dear Ms. ___________,

I am writing as a follow-up to your letter dated [date] regarding care of your daughter, [name], at [name] Medical Center on [date]. We appreciate hearing your opinion as we continually look for ways to improve our services.

We have done an investigation of your daughter's stay with staff responsible for the areas identified in your letter. Thank you for your patience during the last two months awaiting our response. The following responses should hopefully address your concerns.

Wounds from cast removal—This issue is not due to an outdated saw but rather due to a lack of padding on the initial cast (applied at [name of other hospital]). There was only one layer of stockinet and no other padding beneath the cast. This is not the unusual process for applying casts and had Dr. [name] known there was no padding, he could have tried other maneuvers to avoid an injury to the underlying skin. The saw used to cut the cast was not old nor were the blades dull.

Repair of wounds—Since the wounds were superficial and not bleeding, it was decided to dress the wounds and re-cast the arm. Since this was an abrasion from the cast saw itself, there is unfortunately no option to suture a wound or Steri-strip a wound that has been abraded longitudinally the width of the saw blade. It would have required essentially excising the longitudinal abrasion and then closing it up.

Follow-up contact—Although Dr. [name] explained to you what happened following the cast removal, we failed to make formal follow-up contact other than mailing a satisfaction survey form. We apologize for this.

Waterproof cast—[Name] Medical Center does use water proof casting and Dr. [name] does agree that this is a more comfortable option, but he chooses not to use waterproof casting until the fracture has united and is not something he uses routinely on initial casting.

Parental attendance in the x-ray department—The preferred practice at [name] Medical Center is not to allow parents in the exam room during an x-ray. This is done because x-ray staff has seen through their experience that children are more cooperative if the parent is not in the room. Individual situations are taken into consideration when needed. If a parent is allowed in the room, they remain behind the control panel during the exposure, but always having full sight of the child.

Since the time of [name]'s visit, we have acted to improve the communication of this policy to parents by posting a sign in the waiting area.

Cafeteria time—Because we are a small health care facility, we are limited in our kitchen/dining room space. Therefore, we need to close our cafeteria over the noon hour to prepare trays for the hospital patients and nursing home residents. We have added a "Soup & Salad" option on Tuesdays and Thursdays to accommodate visitors and staff while the dietary department is closed. We are looking into possibly expanding this option to another day a week. The vending machines are also available 24 hours a day, which contain microwaveable food items.

We are sorry you were dissatisfied with the above items and hope you accept our responses and/or actions taken to improve some issues. Again, thank you for your letter and we hope you will choose [name] Medical Center for your health care needs if you are in the area.

Sincerely,

[Name]
[Title]

Responding to a case: When the medical staff made an error

Issue: Root cause analysis

Analysis: The following letter addresses medical staff error. It does a good job of validating the complaint, explaining about the process, and detailing how corrective action is being implemented. Further, it is a good example of how to notify dissatisfied patients of their right to address complaints with the Department of Health, as required in some states. The end reassurance about providing future care could be phrased more strongly.

[Date]

[Name]
[Address]

Dear Ms. ______________,

I am writing to follow up on your concerns regarding the care and treatment you received during your recent hospitalization at [name] Hospital. Please accept my apology for the inconvenience of having to perform one procedure two times. The fact that the enema performed on [date] was initiated through the rectum and had to be redone through your colostomy site is not acceptable. Our expectation is that we perform the correct procedure at the correct site every time. We did take the opportunity to learn from this experience in order to improve care for all patients at [name] Hospital.

As promised, we did conduct a root cause analysis to determine where opportunities for improvement exist. A multi-disciplinary group of staff including the medical staff, nursing, nurse practitioners, medical imaging and administration did determine that better communication would decrease the likelihood of this happening again. As a result of this analysis, we are taking active steps to improve how procedures are ordered through our computer system. It is imperative that all providers of health care clearly understand what is ordered and how the order will be followed through. We are also changing the process in which "special instructions" (e.g., through the colostomy site) are conveyed. This information will be shared with the staff through staff meetings and to the medical staff through their monthly newsletter.

Thank you for choosing [name] Hospital as your provider and again, I apologize for your experience. I hope that if we are ever privileged to provide you or your family care in the future that we will exceed your expectations. If I can provide further assistance, please contact me at [telephone number]

Sincerely,

[Name]

(This letter included, as required by its state law, contact information for the Department of Health as well as this brief statement: [state name] Patients Rights legislation preserves your ability to complain to the Department of Health. If you are not satisfied with our review and response to your complaint, you may contact the [state] Department of Health Office of Health Systems Management at [contact information].)

Issue: Surgery with unfavorable outcome—negotiating reasonable compensation

Analysis: This letter takes the "novel approach" mentioned in Chapter 1, "Responding to Patient Complaints: Legal Requirements and Issues." The writer agrees to negotiate compensation without attorneys. It is a good example of following-up a phone call in writing, including a recap of the call and statements made by both parties. It is genial yet businesslike, and manages to take responsibility without admitting culpability.

[Date]

[Name]
[Address]

Dear Mrs. _____________,

This letter is to follow-up our telephone conversation from this morning. I am glad that you returned my call so we could discuss the outcome of your surgery on your wrist. As we discussed you will have your husband mail or fax (please see my contact information below) to me copies of the reports from your neurologist and the hand specialist. Also, I asked that you send me copies of your billing statements for both of these physicians so that I could take care of the bill.

You stated to me that you were maintaining good spirits. Also, that you are participating in physical therapy for your hand and arm and are scheduled to see a hand specialist. You also told me that the neurologist had told you that improvement of the use of your hand was not promising, but that you were willing to continue with the process to ensure as positive an outcome as possible.

Lastly, you stated that you did not want to hire an attorney and hoped that we would be willing to compensate you should you not attain full use of your hand. I do concur with this and we can negotiate a reasonable compensation when you feel that you are ready to do so.

Should you have any questions feel free to contact me at [address], [telephone number], [fax number].

Sincerely,

[Name]
[Title]

Issue: Missed diagnosis

Analysis: This letter misses the good customer service steps that can help prevent escalating an issue. Instead, it is filled with very detailed medical jargon, explicitly states the doctor's error, assigns a level of blame to the complainant, and details corrective action taken. While it is good to share that corrections will be made (when appropriate), this is a somewhat wishy-washy implementation and might be better stated more generally. However, it does do a good job of explaining the process and thus reassuring the patient that the hospital is taking the concern seriously and will work to improve patient care.

[Date]

[Name]

[Address]

Dear Mr. __________,

Thank you for your letter of [date], which related your emergency department experience from [date]. It is unfortunate that the appropriate diagnosis was not made during your visit here.

I shared your letter with Dr. [attending doctor name], Dr. [name], ER medical director, the ER nurse manager and the nurse executive. Dr. [attending doctor name] commented that he saw what appeared to be a small infiltrate in the lower lobe of the left lung, causing him to consider pneumonia. He further stated that since there was no tenderness in the right upper quadrant of the abdomen, he thought that the origin of the pain was gastric or stomach and treatment was targeted toward that diagnosis. Although Dr. [attending doctor name] did not recognize the gallbladder disease, other appropriate diagnosis had been excluded. Had you returned, his follow-up treatment options would have included gall bladder ultrasound and narcotics. In hindsight, Dr. [attending doctor name] stated he could have obtained a consultation with a surgeon, which may have resulted in admission for observation of the pain.

Dr. [name] also reviewed your record and discussed the case with Dr. [attending doctor name]. He commented that he thought process for work-up, diagnosis, and treatment makes sense. The liver enzymes and bilirubin were normal and the location of the pain was not typical for gallbladder disease. He shared two thoughts for the physicians to consider in the future:

1. When able, the attending physician should review x-ray films with the radiologist.
2. The attending physician should communicate the thought process for the diagnosis and treatment with the patient.

This last suggestion is the most difficult, since the physician sees patients at all hours and sometimes with minimal sleep. The nursing staff should be able to provide some assistance in this area.

This does not change the outcome in your case and I apologize for that. I do want you to know that we have taken you letter very seriously. In addition to the individuals listed above reviewing it, it also will go through our quality improvement process. This includes reporting to the medical staff and the board of directors.

It is only by sharing you comments that we know that there is a problem. Should you have any further questions or comments about future service concerns, feel free to contact me at [telephone number].

Sincerely,

[Name]
[Title – in this case, CEO]

Responding to a case: Refusal of treatment and loss

Issue: Patient care and family communication—patient passed away after refusing treatment

Analysis: This letter follows-up a telephone conversation. It is vague on the points discussed. However, it is a very kind and polite letter, and does a good job of explaining the process and improvements.

[Date]

[Name]
[Address]

Dear Mrs. ____________,

I am writing in response to the concerns that you shared with me during our recent telephone conversation regarding the care of your father, Dr. [name] in [date]. First, please accept my condolences on the loss of your father. The loss of a loved one is a difficult experience and I apologize if we caused any undue stress to you or your family during such a difficult time.

I would like to thank you for sharing your thoughts with me. It is from input such as yours that we are able to improve the care provided to all patients at [name] Hospital. As a result of our conversation, I am developing an educational opportunity for all medical/surgical nursing staff in which a case scenario is presented. Managers will then discuss appropriate mechanisms for handling various situations involving patient care and family communication.

I am working with our department of respiratory therapy to establish a plan for therapists to call family members when a patient refuses a respiratory treatment. In addition, I am working with the director of nutritional services to review the current process for obtaining nutritional assessments and continually monitoring patients' dietary intake. It is expected that the improvements we make in these areas will benefit future patients and families seeking care at [name] Hospital.

If I can provide you with further assistance, please contact me at [telephone number].

Sincerely,

[Name]
[Title]

CHAPTER 10

Replies: Power of Attorney, Legal Mediation, Representation and Third-party Intervention

Chapter 10

Replies: Power of Attorney, Legal Mediation, Representation and Third-party Intervention

Introduction

Please carefully read Chapter 1, "Responding to patient complaints: Legal requirements and issues," if you haven't already. This chapter will provide your best guidance to how to handle complex grievances that may involve a legal situation.

Power of attorney

Definition of a power of attorney

A power of attorney is a document that formally creates evidence of a relationship between two people that enables one party to act on the behalf of another, such as making health care decisions.

The two parties are designated as the "principal" and the "agent." The principal designates the agent in the document, and authorizes the agent to act on the principal's behalf for whatever business the power of attorney permits.

Powers of attorney range in degree of the amount of acting an agent may do on behalf of the principal. A general power of attorney may allow the agent to conduct any sort of business on behalf of the principal. A specific power of attorney may limit the agent's authority to transactions specified in the document.

In the health care context, this power of attorney is different from other type of non-health care power of attorney. Note: In this book, power of attorney means health care powers of attorney, that is, those that give an agent the ability to make certain health care decisions on the patient's behalf.

Third parties, such as health care facilities, may treat the agent as if he or she is the principal in any transactions for which the power of attorney grants the agent authority. The hospital will need to see the power of attorney in order to determine what authority the agent has in a health care situation and when to deploy the power of attorney.

Generally, a "durable" power of attorney is necessary for the agent to retain authority once the principal is incapacitated. This is the most common type of power of attorney and is very possibly the type a patient might have with another party. A "durable" power of attorney for health care, for example, provides the agent with the authority managing the principal's health care during the principal's lifetime, regardless of capacity. The distinction, "during the principal's lifetime is important because typically a durable power of attorney is only effective until the principal dies (or the power of attorney is terminated, often by terms stipulate din the power of attorney).

Power of attorney documents are very specific to each individual and jurisdiction. Therefore, you should always seek legal advice from legal professionals about a power of attorney. Hospitals should have a policy for dealing with power of attorney principals and agents and should train staff about this policy.

Power of attorney and the hospital

When presented with a health care power of attorney from a patient, one should look at the power of attorney's format. Is it signed by the patient? Does that signature look like the patient's signature? Is the power of attorney dated? Has it been appropriately witnessed? Has the power of attorney been revoked or is it still in effect? Also, look to whether the agent named in the power of attorney is available to make health care decisions and whether there a "back up" (successor) agent named in case the first agent is unavailable or unwilling. Then, it is very important to look at the content of the health care power of attorney (what the power of attorney actually says) because the terms of the power of attorney will describe the types of powers an agent has and the types of decisions an agent can and cannot make.

Depending on state law (and each state's laws can be different) as well as the terms of a specific health care power of attorney, this type of power of attorney generally describes when the agent will begin to have the powers described in the power of attorney (e.g., when the patient becomes disabled, incapacitated, or incompetent). Until that time or event occurs (see state law for additional criteria), a hospital should communicate with the patient regarding his or her health care. A health care power of attorney can specifically state an agent does not have certain powers (such as regarding withdrawal of life-sustaining treatment), and hospitals should make sure the agent's decisions are consistent with the powers granted to him or her by the patient's power of attorney (check other advance directive documents signed by the patient too). Also, check your state's laws because those laws may describe when a power of attorney is no longer effective and may prohibit an agent from having certain powers, such as regarding sterilization or involuntary commitment.

Many hospitals advise patients and families of power of attorneys upon admission, as part of an admission or registration packet which describes, among other things, the patient's right/opportunity to make advanced directives and the hospital's policy regarding power of attorneys and advanced directives, such as a Do Not Resuscitate or a Living Will (this depends on what types are recognized by your state's laws).

If a patient already has a power of attorney, he or she should bring it to the hospital, and a copy of the power of attorney should be placed in the patient's medical record. If a patient has a power of attorney but left it at home, the patient or family should be instructed to bring the power of attorney to the hospital as soon as practical or the patient can execute a new power of attorney at the hospital. (Note: Some state laws may impose additional requirements for power of attorneys signed while a patient is in a health care facility, such as extra witnesses or special certifications by a physician.)

If a patient has a health care power of attorney, and a circumstance triggering the agent's powers occurs (e.g., the patient becomes comatose and thus is incapacitated), then a physician or hospital can communicate with the agent named in a valid health care power of attorney regarding the patient's health care (but only as to those decisions permitted by the terms of the power of attorney). Risk management and the hospital's lawyer can provide assistance in reviewing the patient's power of attorney and advising health care providers about proceeding with such discussions.

Complaints regarding health care powers of attorney could involve family members who are basically unhappy with the patient's choice as agent (such as in a divorce or step-child situation). Resolution of such complaint may involve explaining that the patient selected this particular agent, and the hospital is merely complying in good faith with decisions made by the agent, in accordance with the patient's power of attorney. Other types of complaints involving power of attorneys could allege the agent is acting outside his powers under the power of attorney, the agent is making a decision contrary to the terms of the power of attorney, or the hospital is improperly relying on a power of attorney, which the family contends has been revoked, altered or is otherwise improper. A hospital receiving such complaints should strongly consider contacting the hospital's lawyer for assistance in reviewing and interpreting the power of attorney, as well as confirming whether the terms of the power of attorney (and the agent's decisions) are consistent with applicable state law.

Issue: Patient's daughter is power of attorney but was not contacted

Background: This letter was sent in response to a complaint from a woman who was angry because the hospital discharged her mother from the emergency department to the care of the person that brought her to the hospital, another daughter and son-in-law. The woman stated that she was the power of attorney and nothing should have been done without consulting her. She did not ever come to the hospital and did not, until requested, provide a copy of the power of attorney document.

[Date]

[Name]
[Address]

Dear _______________

I am writing in response to your complaint of [date], at which time you related your dissatisfaction with how your mother's discharge from care was handled. You also related that as power of attorney, you were denied the ability to make decisions regarding your mother's emergency treatment. Although your complaint was thoroughly investigated by the emergency department director, I was asked to respond to specifically address the issues of health care decision-making and the authority of a power of attorney.

In reviewing the information regarding your mother's emergency department visit, I would note that there is no indication that your mother was incapacitated at any time during the course of her visit to our emergency department. It was noted by multiple health care professionals that your mother was alert, oriented and able to understand the nature of her condition, as well as the treatment options offered. She was further noted to have related that she lived independently in her own home. Your mother demonstrated no behavior, during the course of her stay, which would have lead the health care professionals involved in her care to question her ability to make informed decisions.

The laws pertaining to informed consent and authorized substitute decision-making are clear. Even in the presence of a document designating a power of attorney, the patient does not give up their right to make decisions when they are capable of doing so. This would be the case with your mother. Additionally, in those instances where an incapacitated patient requires emergent intervention, informed consent is implied in the absence of an authorized decision maker. In your mother's case, she was deemed to be competent to make her own decisions and did so. This included her decision to leave the hospital in the company of family other than you.

I hope that this addresses your concerns regarding the treatment your mother received on [date]. It is my understanding that you have provided us with a copy of document assigning you power of attorney. This has been placed in her medical record and should allow for some degree of clarity in the future. However, I would again note that so long as your mother is deemed alert, oriented and capable of making decisions regarding her health care needs, it is our responsibility to honor her right to do so.

Sincerely,

[Name]
[Title]

Legal mediation

There may be times when you refer a situation to your attorney, or the patient refers a situation to his or her attorney. In this case, the documentation of the situation up to this point is crucial, and you should ensure that you carefully document any subsequent communication. Know your hospital's policy and follow it carefully. If all communication is to occur through the attorney's, acknowledge you have received this notice and then conduct all communication only through the attorney as per the terms.

Issue: Patient refers the matter to an attorney

Analysis: This letter acknowledges that the hospital will direct all communication to the complainant's attorney. The strength is that it does this upfront, in a very factual tone. The second paragraph apology and beginning third paragraph reiteration about the hospital's mission are also good to include. However, it probably would have been best to end there and close the letter. When a situation has reached this point, keep your letter short, to the point, and factual.

[Date]

[Name]
[Address]

Mrs. [Name]:

Thank you for your telephone call this week. As you requested, we will now direct all communication and questions concerning your complaints about your son's care to your attorney, [name of attorney], at [mailing and e-mail addresses] and to [phone number].

It is evident from your experience that we did not succeed in exceeding your expectations and for that, I apologize.

We are committed at [hospital name] to creating a caring environment for the families who deliver their children here. Learning about your experience deeply saddens me, yet knowing your perspective helps us find ways to improve our services. The increased awareness provided in our conversation has assisted staff in gaining understanding on better meeting each patient's needs. I am disappointed that we cannot change your experience, but again, I appreciate you taking the opportunity to share your concerns.

If I can provide you with further assistance, please don't hesitate to call me at [telephone number].

Sincerely,

[Name]
[Title]

Issue: Hospital refers the matter to attorney

Note: See Section I, Chapter 2, "HIPAA and Patient Complaints: What to Consider," for more information about the health information privacy complaint.

[Date]

[Name]
[Address]

Dear Mr. ___________________:

This letter is to advise you that any further contact or communication regarding your medical record or your concerns about your emergency room visit, on [date], is to be through your attorney. Please have your attorney direct all correspondence or telephone contacts to the hospital's risk management department. Last week when we again discussed your concerns, the final agreement was that all contact with the Hospital would be through me; therefore, I am writing this letter as a follow-up since you contacted the health records department today.

Multiple department directors and staff have spent a great deal of time trying to meet your needs. You have been provided with copies of your medical record, the medical record policy and forms for amending your medical record. If you wish to amend your medical record please complete them according to the directions supplied to you and send them to the Hospital to the attention of the risk management department.

Acting in conjunction with the Hospital's HIPAA privacy officer, I have enclosed a health information privacy complaint form that was referenced in the "Notice of Denial of Request to Amend Records" that was sent to you by the director of health records services. You may direct your completed form to the Department of Health and Human Services to the attention of [name], [title], [address]. Should you decide to complain to DHHS, you must do so within 180 days from the date of this letter.

Sincerely,

[Name]
[Title]

Enclosure: Health Information Privacy Complaint

Issue: Case is referred to the attorney general

Analysis: The situation this letter addresses (the case was referred to the attorney general) is an excellent example of why it is so important to document. Note how this letter sticks to a factual recitation of details and timelines.

[Date]

[Name]
[Address]

Re:
File #:

Dear Ms.____________,

I am responding to your letter, dated [date], and received by my office on [date]. Attached to your letter was a complaint, filed with your agency by [name of complainant] regarding charges he incurred as a result of seeking treatment in our emergency department.

[Name of complainant] sought care in our emergency department on [date]. At that time he listed [name of insurance] as his insurance carrier. This company was billed [amount] on [date]. Our business office received a call from [name of complainant]'s mother on [date], at which time she indicated that the primary insurance carrier should have been [name of insurance]. This was changed in our system and [name of insurance] was billed on [date]. [Name of insurance] subsequently denied the claim on [date], citing ineligibility for coverage. Based on that denial, the patient was billed [amount] on [date] and again on [date]. On [date], [name of insurance] indicated they would accept the claim. The bill was adjusted based on our contractual agreement with [name of insurance], which reduced the bill to [amount]. [Name of insurance] then submitted payment in the amount of [amount]. The balance of [amount] was billed to the patient on [date], since he had not met his deductible. On [date], [name of complainant]'s mother called and was sent a charity application. A third statement, reflecting a balance due of [amount] was sent on [date]. On [date] an additional statement was sent indicating that the bill would be forwarded to collections within 15 days. We were then notified that a complaint had been filed with your agency.

As you can see, the amount of the bill did not become an issue until it became the patient's responsibility. Any additional adjustment we made would be first refunded back to the insurance company, with the patient responsibility remaining at [amount], which is his deductible.

In addressing the amount of the charges, I would have to respond that the patient sought care in our emergency department. As you are aware, we are required under state and federal law to provide a medical screening examination and appropriate disposition. While I would agree that his condition might well have been treated at a facility other than the emergency department of a level three trauma center, he chose to be seen here. Our charges reflect the costs associated with maintaining the appropriate staffing levels, equipment and technology necessary to respond to a variety of different medical conditions. Although we are prohibited from comparing our prices to those of other hospitals, I am comfortable that our charges fall within the range of usual and customary.

In closing I would point out that through our contractual arrangement with [name of complainant]'s insurance company, [name of insurance], we discounted the charges by twenty-five percent. At this point, I have instructed our business office to re-bill [name of complainant] for the remaining balance of [amount]. We are unwilling to further discount the bill for the services we provided.

Should you require additional information, please do not hesitate to contact me directly at [telephone number].

Sincerely,

[Name]
[Title]

Third-party intervention

The typical third-party intervention is an immediate family member, spouse/significant other or close friend. Many of the other letters demonstrate the large number of mothers, fathers, sons and daughters writing on a patient's behalf. However, sometimes, patients engage a non-family member to speak on their behalf. This third-party intervention may range from a powerful person (such as a senator) to a powerful organization (such as the Department of Health or the Joint Commission on Accreditation of Healthcare Organizations). And, in some other case, it might be a lawyer.

Powerful people

It is important to use the appropriate form of address for the person to whom you are writing. Many people have credentials such as MD, JD, PhD and so forth. The figure below contains guidelines for how to address, open and close letters for some "powerful people" you may need to contact.

Figure 10.1

How to Properly Address a Letter

Although there are no "hard and fast" rules about how to address a letter to important people, there are generally accepted guidelines that are suggested below.

Addressing a letter to a senator

The Honorable (Full Name)
U.S. Senate
Washington DC 20510

Dear Senator (Last Name)

Close with, "Yours respectfully," "Yours sincerely," or "Yours respectfully and sincerely."

Addressing a letter to a representative

The Honorable (Full Name)
U.S. House of Representatives
Washington DC 20515

Dear Congressman or Congresswoman (Last Name)

Close with "Yours respectfully," "Yours sincerely," or "Yours respectfully and sincerely."

Addressing a letter to directors of prisons, police chiefs and local officials including military personnel and judges

Directors of prisons, police chiefs and local officials	Dear Sir/Madam
Military personnel	Dear Admiral/General/Colonel/Captain
Judges	Your Honor

Close with "Yours faithfully."

Figure 10.1

How to Properly Address a Letter (cont.)

Addressing a letter to Archbishops, Cardinals, Bishops, or Vicars/priests

Archbishops	Your Grace
Cardinals	Your Eminence
Bishops	Dear Bishop
Vicars/priests	Dear Reverend/Father

Close with "Yours sincerely."

Addressing a letter when you are unsure about the gender of the person

Dear Sir/Madam, Dear Madam/Sir, or To Whom it May Concern

Addressing a letter to a person with credentials

In the header, use the name and credentials, and then use the credentials and the name in direct address, for example:

[Full name], MD
or
[Full name], PhD

Dear Dr. [Last name]

Addressing a letter—general guidelines for opening and closing the letter

In the header, use the appropriate form of address plus the full name and address. In the beginning of the letter, use Mr. [Last name], Ms. [Last name], or Mrs. [Last name] only. If you are uncertain about a lady's marital status, use Ms. [Last name]. Otherwise, it is appropriate to use Mrs. [Last name] for a married woman. Ensure that you use the correct last name and honor a hyphenated name by using it. The surest way to annoy a person is by getting their name incorrect. Check how the person signed their name on an admission form, for example, to see what name they prefer to use formally. In general, you should not address complainants or their representatives in formal letters by their first name.

Figure 10.1 How to Properly Address a Letter (cont.)

Etiquette states that you should close a business letter using "Yours truly," or "Yours very truly." It is also appropriate to use "Sincerely," "Sincerely yours," "Very sincerely," "Very sincerely yours," "Yours always sincerely," or "Always sincerely yours," for formal letters. In general, it is appropriate to use, "Respectfully" when writing to a customer, or from an employee to an employer, or by an inferior to a superior, never by a person of equal position. Select from any of these, whichever is most comfortable to you or closest to the standard for your organization.

As mentioned in some of the special cases above, "Faithfully" or "Faithfully yours" are appropriate when sending uncommercial correspondence, such as to a dignitary, e.g., a letter to the President of the United States, a member of the Cabinet, an Ambassador, a clergyman, etc. Avoid personal closings, such as, "Warmly," "Best," or "Take care."

Never under any circumstances sign a letter "Mr.," "Mrs.," or "Miss" (except a note written in the third person). Instead sign the letter using your name and credentials, and consider including your title beneath your name.

Issue: Senator intervened on behalf of family—quality of care

[Date]

The Honorable (Full Name)
U.S. Senate
Washington DC 20510

Dear Senator (Last Name),

This is in response to your inquiry on behalf of [name]. Mr. [name]'s son has expressed concerns regarding his father's ongoing care while he was an inpatient at [name of hospital].

Our records indicate that Mr. [name] presented to the emergency room on [date]. He arrived via ambulance after he sustained a fall in his home. Mr. [name] was subsequently admitted for inpatient management of alcohol withdrawal and detoxification placement.

On [date], he was found to be cyanotic, a condition caused by excessive concentration of reduced hemoglobin in the blood. As a result of his condition, he was transferred to the medical intensive care unit for evaluation and management of acute respiratory failure. It was following his stabilization and transfer to a medical unit that Mr. [name] ingested approximately 20 cc of absorbase skin cream. Poison control was contacted and advised that the ingestion was not dangerous.

Mr. [name] exhibited multiple medical failures during his five-month stay at the [name] facility. In addition to his chronic obstructive pulmonary disease his diagnoses included pneumonia, anxiety, sepsis, chest pain, chronic bronchitis, hypertension and asthma.

When the physician staff medically cleared Mr. [name] for discharge, the social worker assisted the family in identifying rehabilitation facilities best equipped to wean Mr. [name] from his ventilator. The family chose[name] as it was in close proximity to the patient's wife.

It was not until shortly before Mr. [name] discharge on [date], that the family voiced their concerns regarding the [date] incident whereby Mr. [name] ingested absorbase cream. Per protocol, they were advised to speak with the patient advocate, [name]. On [date] the patient's daughter called and spoke with Mrs. [name]. The family was requesting the [name] pay for the patient's stay at [name] because of the incident occurring in February. Mrs. [name] advised the patient's daughter of options available to them since the family believed the patient's present condition was a result of this incident. Based on this conversation, the patient's daughter was provided with instructions on pursuing available legal resources.

I hope this information has assisted with questions you may have. Thank you, Senator [name] , for addressing the concerns of Mr. [name]'s family with me.

Sincerely,

[Name]
[Title]

Issue: Senator intervened on behalf of family—patient passed away

[Date]

The Honorable (Full Name)
U.S. Senate
Washington DC 20510

Dear Senator (Last Name),

This is in response to your inquiry on behalf of the family of patient [name]. Mr .[name]'s family has expressed concerns regarding his hospitalization at [name] from [date] to [date].

As a result of your inquiry a member of the Medical Center staff conducted a quality review. The review noted that Mr. [name] is a [age and gender], who was referred to the [name] with an abdominal aortic aneurysm (AAA). He was taken to the Operating Room the day of his admission. He underwent an uncomplicated AAA repair and was transferred to the intensive care unit (ICU), where he was observed. Over the subsequent days, the patient did well and was transferred from the surgical intensive care unit to a surgical patient unit. However, he developed a leukocytosis, a transient increase in the number of leukocytes in the blood, resulting from various causes, as hemorrhage, fever, infection, inflammation, etc. Mr. [name] became increasingly confused without any obvious reason

Mr. [name]'s abdominal exam became increasingly worrisome with marked left lower quadrant tenderness and he underwent a gastric tube placement. It was suspected that the patient most likely had some degree of colonic ischemia and he was taken to the operating room for an exploratory laparotomy on [date]. The findings from this procedure were negative and postoperatively the patient was taken to the ICU. Over the subsequent two weeks Mr.[name]remained intermittently febrile requiring intubation and ventilation. Over the course of treatment Mr. [name]improved, was extubated and was subsequently transferred to the surgical patient unit on [date].

However, on postoperative day 42 Mr. [name] became intermittently febrile again. Following intervention he was again at this postoperative baseline and rehabilitation screening was undertaken. He was accepted to the Rehabilitation Service and was transferred there on June 14, 2002. Sadly, he passed away while an inpatient at [name of hospital] on [date].

I hope this information has assisted with questions you may have. Thank you, Senator [name] for addressing the concerns of Mr. [name]'s family with me.

Sincerely,

[Name]
[Title]

Powerful organizations: Department of Health and JCAHO

Patients may escalate complaints, or at any time, refer complaints to oversight organizations such as the Office for Civil Rights (OCR) or the Joint Commission on Accreditation of Healthcare Organizations (JCAHO). Very commonly, you may be required to refer them and their complaint to the Department of Health (check your state requirements). In these cases, you will need to reply to the organizations that contact you. The following letters are some samples of how you need to respond and information you should include.

Issue: Complaint filed with Department of Health

[Date]

[Name]
[Address]

RE: Complaint #[number]

Dear____________,

I received the complaint filed by Mrs. [name] with the [state] Department of Health concerning the care her husband received at [name] Medical Center on [date]. Upon receipt of the complaint, we contacted [name] and spoke with her by phone. As required, we have also provided her a written response. Enclosed is a copy of that response. Also enclosed is a copy of the procedure reports.

As I know you are aware, the potential for an infection following any invasive procedure is a known risk. Even when there is no known break in sterile technique, as in [patient's name] case, an infection can develop. Our investigation consisted of the following:

- We interviewed the staff involved in [patient]'s procedure and they reported no break in sterile technique or anything out of the ordinary preoperatively, intraoperatively or postoperatively.

- Supplies used in this procedure are for single-use and are disposed of at the conclusion of the procedure. Packaging is routinely inspected prior to use to assure it is intact and in date. There were no problems identified with any of the supplies used.

- We checked the supply inventory in the Cath Lab and all dated items were well within their expiration date.

- We checked with the manufacturer of the Angio-Seal and they reported to us they have had no problems reported.

- We identified 39 patients who had invasive procedures in our Cath Lab the week before, week of and week immediately following [patient]'s procedure. We contacted the physicians of each of these patients to determine whether or not any of them had signs or symptoms of any infection at their follow-up visits. The physicians reported no infections among any of these patients.

Our in-house Infection Control Committee has reviewed our investigative findings and assessed this as an isolated event. We will, however, continue to monitor for any trend or pattern associated with procedures being done in our Cath Lab.

If you need any additional information, please feel free to contact me. We will be happy to provide you any additional information.

Sincerely,

[Name]
[Title]

Issue: Complaint filed with JCAHO

[Date]

[Name]
[Title]
[Address]

Re: Case #

Dear ____________________,

Thank you for bringing this concern to our attention. This letter will explain the outcome of our investigation.

The following are the results of our investigation into the concerns brought to us via your letter, for what appears to be an anonymous complainant:

Our investigation is limited with this complaint since there are no dates, names and specific events. What the investigation did reveal was that we do indeed have a contract with [state] Department of Corrections, but it is to provide medical services to their inmates, and not psychiatric care.

The prison system here has a crisis stabilization program and facility on campus and thus handles psychiatric diagnoses on their own. They are better equipped to provide "suicide watch" for a prisoner than we are. According to the DoC liaison, the only patients we would get here would be those requiring acute medical attention.

As for the patient with the towel around his neck, we have no record of this happening at [location], so we cannot respond to the event without a name and date of incident.

In reference to the 72-hour committal paper work, our facility would provide medical attention to an inmate; however; our psychiatric facility is not physically set up to provide inmate care. Since the commitment papers were mentioned, we know that this must be a local law enforcement agency. DoC provides their own psychiatric services unless psychiatric admission is necessary in which case the inmate is sent to another contracted psychiatric facility down state.

[Name] Healthcare System provides the majority of indigent care for the [region]. We have many patients with no payor resources. It is not our practice to turn patients, any patients away, regardless of payor source.

If we could be provided with names and dates, we could do a chart audit and find out the specific reasons that the patient or patients in question were sent back to the holding facility.

I hope this serves to clarify any questions regarding the validity of these complaints. We are truly saddened that this group of people has the perception that they do, but we are unable to verify that the complaints are valid. We also have no other pending complaints regarding the same sort of issues.

Sincerely,

[Name]
[Title]

CHAPTER 11

Replies: Dealing with Difficult Situations, Difficult People, and Patient Errors

CHAPTER 11

Replies: Dealing with Difficult Situations, Difficult People, and Patient Errors

Introduction

There are situations in which you may find it difficult to formulate a response: perhaps the patient or complainant has been very rude or personally insulting, perhaps the complainant is in error, or perhaps the patient is the problem and so forth. In these cases, it is still important to be polite and professional. This chapter will provide suggestions and guidance to best responses in difficult situations. You'll learn how to

- diffuse anger
- agree to disagree
- respond to patients when the patient is in the wrong

Patrick Donadio[1], a business coach and professional speaker, offers some tips for dealing with people in difficult situations.

The first step is to identify what type of person you're working with and the rationale behind their actions. Understand that you might need to communicate differently with various types of people, he says. The quiet person, for example, might need some advance warning about your meeting and some prompting in order to share ideas. The complainer wants some assurance that his or her voice will be heard and that you'll actually take some action in response.

Following are some tips to help you deal with the many distinct people you encounter:

- Establish some boundaries for yourself. Know what you are going to be able to put up with. Sometimes you might want to communicate those boundaries; sometimes you may not.

- If you're dealing with a difficult issue, speak with the person in private.

---

[1] *Patrick J. Donadio, MBA is a Certified Speaking Professional (CSP) & Master Certified Coach (MCC) who helps leaders and their organizations increase profits, boost performance, improve communications and build better relationships in less time. Visit* www.PatrickDonadio.com *for business tips and more information on his presentations/business coaching. Or call 614/488-9164 or e-mail* Patrick@PatrickDonadio.com.

- Use more "I" language than "you" language, which can a make person become defensive. Instead of saying "you should" or "you must," try "I was expecting" or "I encourage you to…"

- Don't take things personally. "It's hard not to, but it's not necessarily about you," Donadio says. "You need to separate yourself from the issue."

- See if you can find any agreement at all, or at least acknowledge that you understand the person's perspective. Say, "I can see your point." In a worst-case scenario, agree to disagree: "Evidently we both have different opinions on this, and that's OK."

- Tell the person what you can do—not what you can't do—about their request or complaint.

- Rehearse if you need to before communicating a difficult message.

- Keep your cool. If one or both parties start to get upset, suggest resuming the conversation at a later time after you calm down and collect your thoughts.

- Keep the lines of communication open. "Remember that 70 to 90 percent of the message is screened by the receiver," Donadio says. "Ask questions, listen, repeat the problem, restate or rephrase your message," Donadio recommends. "Check for understanding to make sure the message that you sent is the same message the person received."[2]

Diffuse anger

Being in a conflict or disagreement can make your workday very stressful. Additionally, poor handling of the situation can cause it to escalate. Try to identify the complainant's goal in the communication; it may be merely to vent. Figure 11.1 below contains some tips and ideas about how to handle a "complainer." Below Figure 11.1 are sample letters to diffuse anger.

---

[2] *Source: Ohio University Ohio Today Online.* Handle with care: How to deal with difficult people. *By Joan Slattery Wall and Mike Gennaria. Fall 2003* www.ohiou.edu/ohiotoday/fall03/fieldnotes/Donadio/. *Reprinted with permission. Ohio Today Online is a Web site for alumni and friends of Ohio University in Athens, Ohio, and a complement to the university's Ohio Today print publication*

Figure 11.1

The Complainer

Patrick Donadio is a business coach and professional speaker who works in Columbus, Ohio. Donadio has earned the certified speaking professional designation, the highest earned designation awarded by the National Speakers Association, and has been working with business professionals since 1986.

Often, Donadio says, the reason people complain so much is simply because they want to be heard. So, let them complain—for a short while.

"It's important that you acknowledge that you heard what they said," Donadio says. "If you don't acknowledge that you've heard them, they're not going to stop complaining."

Repeat, in your own words, what the person is saying to make sure you've got it right. Next, determine whether there is any legitimacy to the complaint. Then you can move from the problem to the solution.

"You want to get the complainer to take as much ownership as possible," Donadio says. If they can solve the problem on their own, ask for their suggestions. Try to get them to commit to taking action. If it's a problem you have to solve, thank them for bringing it to your attention, ask for ideas and assure them you'll do something about it.

If, on the other hand, the person is complaining simply to complain without any real legitimacy, that is "venting."

"A lot of times just letting them vent for a little bit allows them to feel better," he says. "The biggest thing about dealing with a complainer is not to take it personally."

Source: Ohio University Ohio Today Online. Handle with care: How to deal with difficult people. *By Joan Slattery Wall and Mike Gennaria. Fall 2003.* www.ohiou.edu/ohiotoday/fall03/fieldnotes/Donadio/. *Reprinted with permission. Ohio Today Online is a Web site for alumni and friends of Ohio University in Athens, Ohio, and a complement to the university's Ohio Today print publication.*

Figure 11.2

Hostility Curve

Anger typically follows a cycle.
The key is to not intervene too soon!

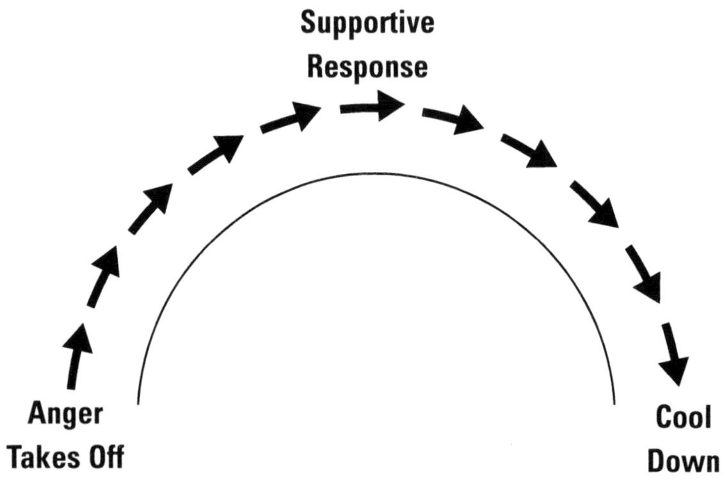

- Call person by name if possible
- Focus on issues, not people
- Voluntarily bring up negatives
- Paraphrase
- Support "venting" but monitor it so it doesn't escalate
- Resist the urge to flee; feeling abandoned can cause the complainant to escalate the situation
- Remember, a complaint is a gift

Source: St. Vincent Charity Hospital, Cleveland, OH. Cindy Ebner, MSN, RN, Director of Risk Management. Reprinted with permission.

Issue: Diffusing a patient's anger

[Date]

[Name]
[Address]

Dear ________,

I am writing to acknowledge that we received your concerns regarding the care [you/name of patient] received at [name of hospital] on [date]. I was very sorry to hear that your experience with us was less than satisfactory.

We take all concerns seriously because our mission is to provide quality care to every patient. We appreciate that you took the time to bring this issue to our attention.

I have looked in to each of the issues that you identified and I have shared your comments with the [department(s) name] director so that appropriate actions may be taken.

Thank you for bringing these issues to our attention. Although we cannot change the experience that you had with us, your observations and comments will help us in our continuing efforts to improve the care that we provide. We hope, that should the need arise, you will allow us the privilege of serving you again in the future.

Sincerely,

[Name]
[Title]

Issue: Sending a conciliatory letter

[Date]

[Name]
[Address]

Dear ____________,

As Director of Performance Improvement for [name of hospital], your letter of [date] detailing your concerns about your care has been referred to me. I thank you for offering your recollections and criticisms of your care and I am grateful that you have taken the time and effort to inform us about your experience.

I believe your comments are valid and deserve a response. Service quality is extremely important at [name of hospital] and we are happy that you gave us the opportunity to follow up on your experience. While it is disappointing that you were dissatisfied with several aspects of your care, such letters are very important to us because they offer an opportunity to see how others view us. Ultimately, we hope that each and every letter of complaint may lead to improvement in the care we render at [name of hospital].

There is no doubt that you suffered through a very trying and difficult time during your hospitalization. The experience had to have been most stressful, beyond what can be expressed in words. Let me assure you that we believe all patients, families and visitors should be treated with respect and dignity and that each patient is afforded the highest level of care possible.

[Consider including a brief description of programs at the hospital and how they should address this concern in the future.]

Patient satisfaction is very important to [name of hospital] and to the staff. Through staff meetings, in-services and staff supervision, we are working with the staff to heighten their awareness of how patient care is perceived and to be more sensitive and responsive to patients' needs.

Once again, we thank you for your letter and we are sorry we did not meet your expectation.

Sincerely,

[Name]
[Title]

Agreeing to disagree

There may be situations in which your response or solution to a situation is unsatisfactory to a patient. For example, a patient may refuse advised treatment, want you to dismiss disputed charges when there is no merit to dismiss, etc. In these cases, continue your polite and professional response, remind the patient of the policy behind the decision, and reiterate that the decision is final. In some states, you may need to let the patient know that he or she may pursue the matter with the Board of Health so make sure you know your state's requirements. In some cases, you may need to let the patient know future communication needs to go through a legal party such as your facility's attorney. Whatever happens, document the course of action and reasons behind it. Keep in mind that the goal of documentation is to protect from vulnerability.

Following are some good samples of agreeing to disagree. Regardless of the different situations they address, the bottom line is that the hospital is unable to comply with the complainant's requested course of action. It is important to communicate this and why while remaining polite and professional. Keep in mind the following tips about dealing with difficult people:

- Each person has a point of view that is valid to that person
- While your points of view may be different, it is okay
- Validate both perspectives and reiterate the decision and basis for the decision

Issue: No reimbursement for lost personal items

[Date]

[Name]
[Address]

RE: [Subject line and/or case number]

Dear ______________,

Your complaint and demand for payment for lost pajama bottoms has been referred to me for review. Based on the information contained within the file, you were brought to our emergency department from a skilled nursing facility where you were recuperating from valve replacement surgery. Following a stay of approximately two (2) hours, you were transferred to [name of hospital] for admission.

During the course of your stay in our emergency department, your pajama bottoms were removed. They were placed in a plastic bag as they were soiled and upon your transfer to another facility did not accompany you. The bag was subsequently disposed of as we do not have facilities to launder or store soiled items.

At this time I must decline to reimburse you in the amount of $50.00 because it is not our practice to reimburse for clothing that is damaged or disposed of in the course of providing emergency treatment. I must also inform you that we do not have the liberty of writing off or adjusting Medicare co-pays, as this is in violation of federal law.

I apologize if there has been any lack of clarity regarding this issue.

Sincerely,

[Name]
[Title]

Issue: Physician refuses to prescribe medication

[Date]

[Name]
[Address]

Dear ______________,

Dr. [name of physician] referred your complaint to me. I am the [title] and it is my job to [state job, e.g., help arbitrate patient dissatisfaction]. I would like to take this opportunity to explain to you in writing why Dr. [name] is unwilling to refill your Phenobarbital prescription.

Dr. [name] has been your physician for [state years]. It is his and our hospital's obligation to provide the highest quality care for our patients. To that end, we must follow the best-known medical care and state and federal law. Dr. [name]'s reasons for refusing to fulfill your prescription are consistent with this and we will not override this decision as you requested. The following are his stated reasons for not refilling your prescription and we are in agreement that this is best care:

- He is concerned that you have not faced your dependence upon alcohol
- Your alcoholism has caused convulsions at one time
- A neurologist has prescribed Phenobarbital to for the prevention of the convulsions, provided that you continue your abstinence from alcohol
- However, you resumed drinking alcohol and are currently exceeding the prescribed doses of Phenobarbital to control your morning shakes in order to be able to go to work
- You have not been keeping your appointments with Dr. [name] for the last [state time] and have requested refills of Phenobarbital over the telephone
- Dr. [name] has warned you that you are abusing both alcohol and Phenobarbital and has warned you about the health risk this poses, including but not limited to irreparable damage to your liver, brain and body in general
- Dr. [name] has stated that he would be grossly negligent to condone such treatment

We want you to know that both [name of hospital] and Dr. [name] wish to help you in all ways possible. However, we wish to treat your disease, not facilitate it. Dr. [name] urges you to admit yourself to a detoxification center immediately.

As I stated, Dr. [name]'s decision is consistent with our policy and best medical practice. Therefore, it is our final decision to not override his decision.

We hope you follow Dr. [name]'s advice for seeking treatment and extend to you our wishes for success.

Sincerely,

[Name]
[Title]

Communicating with a patient when the patient is in the wrong

There will be times when a patient has what seems like an erroneous complaint or a delivers the complaint in an insulting manner. There may be situations in which you must communicate with a patient who is "abusing" the medical care options your facility offers, including attempting to gain medication to abuse and being insulting or assaulting staff. Even in these cases, it is important to remain professional and focus on policy. The following two letters demonstrate how to address complicated situations such as these in a professional manner that protects the hospital.

Issue: Patient refused treatment, demanded prescriptions, and abused staff

[Date]

[Name]
[Address]

Dear ___________,

It was recently brought to my attention that you were dissatisfied with some of the care you received and communication with our staff during your hospitalization from [dates]. [Name of hospital] strives to provide quality care while being sensitive to our patients' needs. I am sorry if you felt this was not your experience.

Concerns regarding your plan of care, including your refusal of essential medical treatment and tests, and your demands for narcotics, were brought to me by members of your health care team, including the medical staff. I understand, and indeed, [name of hospital], endorses, the patients' right to refuse medical treatments. However, we also recognize and endorse the importance of adequately and appropriately caring for our patients. By refusing all medical tests, treatment and care except for specific narcotics, the health care team is unable to provide you with appropriate care.

If you choose to return to [name of hospital] in the future, you need to know that it will be the physicians who guide your medical care through assessments, treatments and medications as appropriate to your diagnosis and condition. I want to clearly communicate to you that by refusing medical treatment that is essential to the treatment of your diagnosis and conditions, the physicians and hospital have the right to discharge you from care if you are medically stable or to transfer you to another medical facility for treatment.

I also have been informed of your continual and repeated abuse of the nursing staff and other members of the health care team. It has been noted that in recent past hospitalizations, you have both verbally and physically abused the nursing staff as well.

While I respect the fact that we all, as individuals, have the right to self expression, I need to inform you that physical and verbal abuse of any staff member at [name of hospital] is unacceptable and will not be tolerated. We value each of our employees and are committed to maintaining a safe environment for them, just as we are committed to the safety of our patients.

As a provider of care, we are committed to delivering the best quality and most appropriate medical care that we can, and we want to be responsive to your individual needs. What we cannot do, [name of patient], is to compromise your care or the safety of our staff in the process. I can assure you that [name of hospital] will serve your health care needs, as determined by your treating physicians, should you choose to return to our facility for care.

Sincerely,

[Name]
[Title]

Issue: Patient expresses prejudice and bigotry

[Date]

[Name]
[Address]

Dear ____________,

It was recently brought to my attention that you experienced some inconvenience during your hospitalization from [dates]. I would like to extend my apologies that you needed to be moved from your original room due to facilities issues. I know that making a move of that nature was an inconvenience for you and want to assure you that our engineering staff works hard to try to prevent those types of occurrences.

I also have been informed of your request that specific staff members, particularly those of Philippine descent, not be allowed to participate in your care here at [name of hospital]. While I respect the fact that we all, as individuals, are entitled to hold to our own beliefs and opinions, I need to inform you that [name of hospital] is an equal opportunity employer. As such, we not only employ individuals from a broad spectrum of cultural, ethnic and racial backgrounds, but also we value the individual contributions that each of those individuals makes to our success as an organization.

It is my understanding that during the aforementioned hospitalization, our staff altered their assignments to accommodate your request not to be cared for by Filipino staff members. Please be advised that in the future we will not accommodate a request to exclude staff from your care on the basis of race, ethnicity, cultural background or any other protected class. If this is unacceptable to you, you will need to find another health care institution.

As a provider of care, we are absolutely committed to delivering the best possible medical care that we can, and we want to be responsive to your individual needs. What we cannot do, [name of patient], is show any level of disrespect to our own staff in the process. We employ individuals who are skilled and competent to provide care to every one of our patients. I can assure you that your health care needs will be taken care of with the utmost professionalism.

Sincerely,

[Name]
[Title]

Responding to inquiries from significant others with no recognized legal relation

Responding to complaints or inquiries from a person with no recognized legal authority to intervene for a patient can be a touchy issue. You must comply with privacy regulations but still be tactful. Rather than telling the person what you can't do, follow the tips from this chapter and explain how you can help. The following letter is a good example of how to address this. The representative contacted the patient directly, expressed a desire to cooperate, and explained the steps the patient can take to allow the hospital to communicate with a third-party. This demonstrates respect for the two people and their situation.

Issue: Patient's significant other wants to participate in care

[Date]

[Name]
[Address]

Dear Mr. _______________,

I spoke today with your significant other, ___________. At the time of his phone call, Mr. ___________ expressed concern about your medical condition and wished to discuss the care you had received at Hospital. I explained to Mr._____ that state and federal laws preclude me from disclosing confidential patient information without your written consent. He indicated that you would consent to our discussing your condition with him and, in fact, had signed a release for him to receive medical information.

Following my brief conversation with Mr. ________, I checked with our medical records department and there was no signed release contained within your record. Based on the lack of a signed authorization for release of information, I am unable to provide Mr. ________ with information regarding your condition or the care you received at our facility. Should you desire for him to have access to your confidential health care information, I am forwarding a form for your signature and completion. Once I have received the completed form, I would be happy to speak with Mr. ________ or any other individual you might designate.

With regard to my conversation today, I would note that Mr. ________ related that you were continuing to have what he described as "seizures." He was at a loss as to why they would prescribe a heart medication for a neurological condition. As you are well aware, you have received an extensive work-up both here and in [name of facility]. Your previous work-up in [name of facility] indicated that your "seizures" were likely attributable to cardiac rhythm problems and not your brain. This is why [name of drug]was prescribed then and during your most recent hospitalization.

At the time of discharge on late [date], you were instructed to arrange for a "sleep EEG" and to follow-up with your primary care provider. If you have not done this, you should arrange for the follow-up and testing immediately. If the medication prescribed is found to be no longer effective, there may be other medications that your primary care physician can provide.

In closing I must again encourage you to proceed with arrangements for follow-up care with your primary care provider. Should you wish for me to provide Mr. ________ with information regarding your care and/or condition, please complete the form and return it to me as soon as possible. You may contact me directly with any questions or concerns at [telephone number].

Sincerely,

[Name]
[Title]

SECTION IV

HOW TO RESPOND TO INTERNAL GRIEVANCES

SECTION IV CONTENTS

CHAPTER 12

Allowing for, Processing, and Responding to Employee Concerns

Chapter 12

Allowing for, Processing, and Responding to Employee Concerns

Introduction

A hospital's staff may be the best resource for determining where performance needs improvement and how to minimize risk. Staff are typically up-to-date on requirements, and deal directly with the patients; they observe and can identify areas that may cause complaints. Take advantage of this resource and make staff feel comfortable sharing concerns. Encourage staff to share concerns and ideas, and provide the necessary means for them to do so. Then, make sure to create a way to respond to the complaints and measure the effectiveness for improvements.

If you help handle employee complaints, you can help improve your overall service to patients and families, and create a better environment and improve staff morale. If your staff is unhappy about the quality of care or service, and their complaints are not addressed, they could become a threat to your institution. There have been many government cases in which prosecutors relied on the testimony of "inside" whistleblowers (former hospital employees) to prove their cases.

Some ideas include the following:

- Select an employee or group of employees who will be responsible for passing along overheard comments or concerns.
- Respond to employee complaints concerning quality of care and other important issues. Well-established procedures for addressing worker concerns may reduce or eliminate situations in which patients will complain.
- Keep records of employee concerns and check in at regular intervals to ensure that the problem has been addressed and is no longer an issue.
- Consider allowing employees to share concerns anonymously.
- Communicate that the facility welcomes feedback and there is no repercussion to sharing an honest concern.

- Treat employees who are sharing concerns with the same courtesy you would a patient: validate the concern, investigate if necessary, respond, etc.

- Be prepared to enlist the aid of and cooperation of managers if the concern is a legitimate area that needs performance improvement.

- If an employee precipitates a necessary change and/or assists in performance improvement, make sure to reward that employee. This will encourage future employee participation.

The following two letters are good examples of taking employee concerns seriously and using the same good customer service techniques with employees as with patients. The first letter (memo) does an excellent job with reassuring the employee that they did the right thing, and then providing as much detail as possible for each issue.

Issue: Employee is concerned about quality of care in radiology

MEMO

To: [Name]
From: [Name]
Date: [Date]
Re: **Employee concerns regarding [Name] Healthcare Network**

First, I'd like to thank you for bringing your concerns to my attention. I strongly believe that you did the right thing and that your concerns come from true dedication and commitment to [Name]. I'd like to address each of your concerns one at a time:

Radiation Oncology Equipment
The radiation oncology department owns two machines to administer radiation. One of the machines experienced technical difficulty recently and was not operating. The problem has been corrected and both machines are operating properly. However, there is a severe shortage of radiation technologists, not only at [Name] ([name]), but throughout the health care industry. Due to this staffing crisis, [name] has been forced to close one machine until a qualified radiation technologist can be hired. I understand that the department is currently interviewing potential candidates.

[Other facility]
I spoke with the employee health coordinator regarding the issue you raised about [other facility] sending a patient to a non-[name] facility. The coordinator indicated that there was likely a specific reason that the patient visited a non-[name] facility. It is policy that any employee who visits [other facility] and requires a follow-up visit is directed to an [name] panel of physicians. Without knowing the specifics of this situation, she was unable to provide any reason why this employee may have been directed to a non-[name] facility.

Departure of Long-Term Physicians
I spoke with human resources regarding your concern of long-term physicians departing [name]. There are several factors related to the departure of some of these physicians. First, due to the current malpractice crisis in Pennsylvania, many physicians are being forced to take their practices to other states, where malpractice insurance rates are not as high. Our geographic location in Philadelphia makes us uniquely susceptible to physicians departing for New Jersey and Delaware. The malpractice crisis has hit orthopedists, surgeons, and OB/GYNs particularly hard.

Human resources also informed me that some physicians' contracts were terminated this year. In many of the situations, [name] had to cut losses due to low patient volumes in some specialty areas.

[name] is looking to build its business in some specialties, while recognizing that we are unable to compete in other specialty areas. Recently, Pennsylvania eliminated a Certificate of Need law. This law required that all health care organizations that wanted to add a new service had to apply through the state to build that service. The state reviewed these applications to determine whether or not the service was needed based on population and illness statistics. Now, health care organizations can build whatever service they want, basically unchecked. This means that competition is greater in many specialties.

Physicians Sending Patients to Other Hospitals
In some cases, we work in partnership with other area facilities to offer services that are not currently offered through [name]. Although I am unable to specifically address the situation regarding the physician you identified, I can respond to other instances of physicians sending patients to other hospitals. I am aware that some voluntary (non-[name] employed) physicians have been sending patients to other facilities due to perceived difficulty with admitting patients to [name]. During the past several months, there have been much higher patient volumes than anticipated, contributing to fewer available beds. This has caused delays in admitting patients from the ER and directly from physician offices into inpatient beds. Administration recognized this concern several months ago and began to develop strategies to address this situation. In September, [name] will open a new 16-bed Admissions Unit, which will help to improve the admissions flow from the ER and physician offices. Voluntary physicians are currently being educated about the new unit and we hope to persuade them to continue to send patients to our facility.

Long Waits for Appointments
As discussed, there is currently a "Wait Times" subcommittee that is addressing the wait time to make an appointment through [appointment scheduler telephone number]. Administration is aware of this problem and will continue to monitor the situation and make every improvement necessary to eliminate this wait time.

Staffing Ratio
As discussed, [name] would never put its patients in any kind of jeopardy by having fewer staff than required. We have several staffing agencies that supply us with temporary help when there are too few caregivers available to care for our patients. The health and safety of our patients is our number one concern.

I hope that I have been able to sufficiently address your concerns. Again, I truly appreciate your bringing these issues to my attention and encourage you to continue to voice your concerns. It is only by awareness that we can work to improve our patients' well-being.

Issue: Physician concerned about care of patient

[Date]

[Name]
[Address]

Dear Dr. ____________________ ,

I just wanted to let you know that I visited Mr. [name] earlier today and spent some time with him to learn more about his experience here last night. He indicated that for the most part, his care has been very good. However, there was a gap in service last night. His main concern was timeliness of staff to address his care needs. I spoke with the nurse manager on [name of floor], who indicated that she would personally speak with Mr. [name] and ensure that he had staff appropriately attending to his needs this evening and through the night. She will also inform the clinical manager of Mr. [name]'s needs. I will also personally visit Mr. [name] again at the end of the day to ensure that he is satisfied with the care he has received today.

I also informed the Director of Patient Services about Mr. [name]'s concerns. She and her staff (patient advocates) will continue to visit Mr. [name] throughout the day today, tonight and tomorrow. I will unfortunately be out tomorrow, so her staff will ensure that Mr. [name]'s needs are attended to and that he is comfortable.

Thank you for bringing this matter to my attention. If you have any additional concerns, please don't hesitate to contact me at [telephone number].

Best,

[Name]
[Title]

Section V

Guide to Responding

Section V Contents

Chapter 13

What Not to Write

Chapter 13

What Not to Write

Introduction

There are several symptoms of a bad letter; each of the following could cause the complaint to fester, lead to another complaint, or provide the patient or family with evidence to file a lawsuit:

- Avoid templates. Although it's okay to start with a template for certain types of letters, they don't uphold patient customer service efforts and patients today see right through the "form" letter style. They could lead to miscommunication that creates further complaints.

- Watch for letters that lack details. Detailed letters document the situation for your institution, and they clarify the situation for the complainant, thus potentially saving you time. If you spend a few extra minutes writing a letter, it will save time on the back end, perhaps writing another letter or handling a phone call from the patient, who's now more confused.

- Keep emotion out of it. Don't react personally. And don't communicate in a manner or with information that may make the hospital vulnerable. But when you inject opinions you put your hospital at risk. Make sure to read Chapter 1, "Responding to Patient Complaints: Legal Requirements and Issues," to learn more about risk and get tips about how to address it.

For additional information about what you need to know about responding to grievances, you may want to review the chapters in Section I.

Using many words to say nothing

The key when a mistake is made to express apology but do so without admitting culpability.

Limit your details to the facts only and overarching result of your findings.

Make sure that you are to the point in your letter and include necessary details and an appropriate expression of sympathy, validation, etc. Then, end the letter. Repetition and using many words to say nothing may annoy or confuse a complainant, and worst of all, unintentionally signal that you are not taking the matter seriously. This may cause the complainant to escalate the situation.

Documenting a phone conversation but without any detail

The following letters have the right idea: following up on a phone conversation with a letter. Unfortunately, the letter shares no details or information. For the hospital, this can be an issue in two main ways. First, the purpose of the letter is to reiterate in writing the agreement and information discussed verbally. It can be difficult to recall exactly who said what and this can lead to misunderstanding. In the letter, briefly review the major points of the conversation. Second, this letter is an important piece of the "paper trail" of documentation for all complaints. Make sure a week from now—or a year from now—you or a coworker has enough information in each letter to know the exact situation.

The first letter is the original. The second letter contains fictional additional information to demonstrate how it should be written.

Original

[Date]

[Name]
[Address]

Dear ____________,

I am writing in follow-up of our most recent conversation. As both Dr. [name] and I have informed you, your concern has been taken seriously and an investigation has been done.

I appreciate you sharing your concerns and am hopeful that the information I gave you today will be helpful in identifying those individuals you should ask for if you have a need for assistance regarding your care. Again, if you should have a concern in the future, I encourage you to bring your concern forward so it can be addressed at the time.

Please feel free to call me at [telephone number] if I can be of any further assistance. If you do not feel your concerns have been addressed satisfactorily, please feel free to contact the State Department of Health in [City] at [telephone number].

Sincerely,

[Name]
[Title]

Rewrite

[Date]

[Name]
[Address]

Dear ______________,

I appreciate you sharing your concerns [state method and date of original communication] about your experience while receiving care in our hospital. I am writing in follow-up of our most recent conversation on [date]. As both Dr. [name] and I have informed you, we have taken your concern seriously and we completed an investigation. To briefly recap what we discussed on the telephone, the results of the investigation and action taken are:

- The nurse did not respond to your call in a timely manner. It is our policy that the assigned nurse should respond to a patient's call in [department] within [number] of minutes. We concur with you that the three incidents in which the nurse instead took three times that amount ([number] of minutes) is unacceptable.

- We identified a part of the response process that could be improved. We have since altered the process to better enable nurses to respond within a timely manner. We have also spoken to the nurses to reiterate the importance of responding to all calls.

If you are ever in the same position again, please do not hesitate to bring forward your concerns. When patients like you communicate issues such as this, it is incredibly helpful to us so that we may continuously meet expectations of care and improve quality of care. As I mentioned, you may contact me directly, or contact [name and title] or [name and title].

If you do not feel your concerns have been addressed satisfactorily, please feel free to contact the State Department of Health in [City] at [telephone number].

Sincerely,

[Name]
[Title]

Original

[Date]

[Name]
[Address]

Dear ____________,

I am writing in reference to our phone conversation regarding your husband's [date] hospitalization.

I appreciate you sharing your concerns and assure you that they have been addressed and follow-up has been completed. I hope knowing this is reassuring to you. I realize this must be a very difficult time for you and your family. Thank you for taking the time to talk with me. If I can do anything further, please feel free to contact me at [telephone number]

As with any concern brought to our attention, if you do not feel that they have been adequately addressed, please feel free to contact the State Department of Health in [City] at [telephone number].

Sincerely,

[Name]
[Title]

Rewrite

[Date]

[Name]
[Address]

Dear ________________,

I am writing in reference to our telephone conversation on [date] regarding your husband's [date] hospitalization.

I appreciate you sharing your concerns. I want to assure you that we consider your concerns valid. As we discussed, it is our hospital's policy to support as best as we can the family members of critically ill patients. I passed along your suggestions that the hospital acquire additional cots. [Name], our hospital's [title], also has met with the nurses involved. They discussed better ways to ask family members to move so they can care for the patient.

I hope knowing this is reassuring to you. I realize this must be a very difficult time for you and your family. Thank you for taking the time to talk with me. If I can do anything further, please feel free to contact me at [telephone number]

As with any concern brought to our attention, if you do not feel that they have been adequately addressed, please feel free to contact the State Department of Health in [City] at [telephone number].

Sincerely,

[Name]
[Title]

Resolving without details is no resolution

As with the letters that followed-up phone calls, the following two letters have the right idea: documenting and responding to a complaint. However, one of the most important methods of validating a concern is to repeat the concern. Neither letter states the concern. Restating the concern demonstrates that the hospital heard and understood the concern. Additionally, these letters are so devoid of details that they lack the personal touch that reassures the patient. It's important to let patients know in every communication what your hospital's policy or mission is regarding their specific concern. Further, the lack of detail prevents the hospital from having adequate documentation of the issue.

The first letter is the original. The second letter contains fictional additional information to demonstrate how it should be written.

Original

[Date]

[Name]
[Address]

Dear ____________________,

This letter is in response to your concerns regarding your care by one of our physicians during your emergency department (ED) visit. I have reviewed the complaint and asked a physician to also review the care you received. The investigation included a review of the medical record and discussion with the physician involved. We apologize for your experience and would like to inform you that every complaint is investigated thoroughly. Our expectations of the professional care received by our patients is that it is satisfactory to them.

Thank you again for bringing your concerns to our attention. If you have any questions please feel free to contact our department at [telephone number].

Sincerely,

[Name]
[Title]

Rewrite

[Date]

[Name]
[Address]

Dear ____________________,

I am writing this letter in response to your concerns [state method and date of original communication] regarding the care you received from one of our physicians during your emergency department (ED) visit. You expressed concern about receiving tests without explanation. You communicated that you would have liked to be better informed about the tests you were receiving. We understand that patients like to know what each diagnostic test is and why they are being tested. It is our goal to communicate with patients and answer all of their questions respectfully. I apologize that you did not receive this standard of care.

I have reviewed the complaint and asked a physician to also review the care you received. The investigation included a review of the medical record and discussion with the physician involved. We found that the tests you received were appropriate to the symptoms you presented with. I hope that your additional conversation with Dr. [name] in which he detailed [name tests] that you received answered your questions. Please feel free to call Dr. [name] if you have any further questions.

The director of our ED spoke to the physician involved. The director reminded the physician that it is our policy to respectfully answer all patient questions.

We apologize for your experience. We expect that our patients receive professional care that is satisfactory to them.

Thank you again for bringing your concerns to our attention. If you have any questions please feel free to contact our department at [telephone number].

Sincerely,

[Name]
[Title]

Original

[Date]

[Name]
[Address]

Dear _______________,

This letter is written in response to your concerns regarding your mother's care by one of our physicians during her admission. Dr. [name], the chief of medical services, and I have reviewed the complaint. The investigation included a review of the medical record and discussion with the physician involved. We apologize for your experience and would like to inform you that every complaint is investigated thoroughly through our expectations of professional behavior from all of the physicians on staff.

Please accept our apology for the difficulties your family experienced during her recent hospitalization at [name] Medical Center.

Sincerely,

[Name]
[Title]

Rewrite

[Date]

[Name]
[Address]

Dear ____________________,

This letter is written in response to your concerns [state method and date of original communication] regarding your mother's care by one of our physicians during her admission. We understand that your concerns specifically were [state issues].

Dr. [name], the chief of medical services, and I have reviewed the complaint. Our investigation included reviewing the medical record and discussing the case with the physician involved. The results of our investigation are:

- [specify finding point-by-point for each stated concern]
  We apologize for your experience. Our hospital's mission emphasizes quality of care and we strive to ensure that every patient's care meets or exceeds his or her expectations.

Please accept our apology for the difficulties your family experienced during your mother's recent hospitalization at [name] Medical Center.

Sincerely,

[Name]
[Title]

Taking it too personally: Responding politely to angry situations

Patients may not always complain in a courteous and polite manner. It's difficult to accept this—and possibly worse behavior such as personal insults—when it is directed at you or is about a coworker you know and respect. It may be especially difficult when you fear the repercussions for yourself or your coworker.

However it is integral to set that aside and conduct all communications in a polite and professional manner that is consistent with hospital policy. Ask a colleague in risk management to do a "polite check" of your letter or hand off the job to a colleague. Consider a draft response, doing another task for a while, then return to the draft at a later time when you can be more objective. If all else fails, if possible, consider passing the situation along to a colleague.

The letter below does not follow the guidelines in Figure 13.1 for how to best respond to a patient. It uses many "you" statements and does not validate the complaint. In fact, it does the opposite. This letter is not the sort that will diffuse and resolve a situation; it is the sort of letter that might, in fact, prompt the patient to escalate the complaint, refuse to seek treatment at your hospital in the future, or cause others to avoid your facility after hearing this story. This is not good for the hospital or your time, even if the complaint is not one that will, for example, result in disciplinary measures.

Figure 13.1

Good and Bad Customer Service

When a patient comes to you for assistance, how do you help him/her? Do you listen attentively to what your patient has to say (or what he or she writes) before jumping to conclusions? Do you have the accurate knowledge needed to guide the patient to proper sources of information? Do you have a pleasant and helpful attitude regardless of how you feel at the moment?

10 Points of good customer service include the following:

- Listening carefully first to the patient or read the patient's letter before providing any assistance.
- Thinking from your patient's perspective to understand your patient's concern(s).
- Analyzing your patient's question and determining the root problem(s) he/she faces.
- Keeping yourself up-to-date and educated with the latest knowledge in order to provide your patient accurate and current information.
- Explaining information clearly, concisely, and courteously.
- Respecting your patient, being patient and sympathetic, being aware of the fact that the complexity of hospital rules, administration and policies may be difficult to understand.
- Finding, or if requested, transferring the patient to the proper source of information. Directing your patient to proper sources of information.
- Making the extra efforts necessary to obtain the information for the patient and get back to the patient with the correct information as soon as possible if you do not have the information readily available.
- Maintaining a positive, pleasant attitude regardless of your mood at the moment.
- Constantly reminding yourself of your ultimate purpose—serving the patients and fulfilling the hospital's mission.

10 Points of bad customer service include the following:

- Speaking too soon or interrupting the patient before he or she is done speaking. Speaking unclearly (e.g., mumbling, speaking with your head turned away, or talking too fast) and expecting your patient to understand.
- Focusing on your perspective and ignoring your patient's feelings.
- Assuming you know what the problem is and dealing with the surface issue without trying to find out the real reason the patient is contacting you.
- Not keeping up-to-date with the latest knowledge and information.
- Writing a letter with insufficient detail.
- Expecting your patient to understand the hospital rules, administration and policies.
- Making up information if you do not know the answers to your patient's questions.
- Not going the extra mile to help your patient to obtain the information he/she needs.
- Behaving rudely or arrogantly to your patient, especially when you are having a bad day.
- Talking negatively about patients; consider how this affects your view of patients and how you influence others around you and their view about the patients.

Source: Based on a lesson at http://199.211.83.208/public/lesson12/good.html. *William Winkenwerder, Jr., M.D., M.B.A., Assistant Secretary of Defense for Health Affairs, Executive Director, TRICARE Management Activity. TRICARE University (TRICARE U) is a distance-learning vehicle designed to offer online courses about the various aspects of the TRICARE program and the TRICARE Management Activity (TMA).*

Try to keep in mind that every complaint is an opportunity for performance improvement. Perhaps the improvement in the following letter's situation is to ensure that all patients have their expectations set for how the emergency department works and that there is likely to be a wait.

Additionally, it is not appropriate to judge a complaint as valid or invalid. Limit your response to validating the complaint, discussing hospital policy, and explaining how the problem will be resolved.

And lastly, each complaint is an opportunity for patient service performance improvement. If someone's anger seems out of proportion to the situation, there might be an additional underlying issue. You might have to ask a few questions to get to the true issue and to best understand what the real problem is. In this sample letter, it is clear that the patient expressed anger about a variety of situations, but the key is that she found the physician "disrespectful and uncompassionate." Rather than dismissing this complaint because it is not a common complaint about this physician, the writer should have attempted to delve into what this phrase meant to the patient and how she would have preferred to be treated.

Following are some sample letters. The first letter is the original. The second letter contains fictional additional information to demonstrate how it should be written.

Original

[Date]

[Name]
[Address]

Dear____________,

Your complaint and demand for retraction of your bill was forwarded to me by [name], director of emergency services, for review.

Based on my review of the information contained within your letter as well as information obtained from the medical record and treatment providers, it would appear that you arrived at our emergency department at [date and time] with complaints of [symptoms] for approximately three days. As required by law, you were assessed and found to have stable vital signs. At that point you would be asked to register and it is likely, as you indicated, that you would not be sent immediately back to the an examining room. While we do seek to provide care in an expeditious manner, we do so by severity of condition. If a patient came in after you and was determined to have a condition that was more serious, they would be seen before you.

Our records do indicate that you were examined, specimens were sent to the lab and a course of treatment was formulated and prescribed. You were discharged at [time], two hours and 19 minutes from the time you were checked in. This is not an unreasonable amount of time for treatment received in an emergency room.

With regard to your additional complaints, I am sorry that your perception of the care provided by Dr. [name] was that he was "disrespectful and uncompassionate." Those are not words that I have ever heard used in describing his practice. His professionalism is confirmed by staff members and colleagues alike.

In your letter to Mrs. [name, dated [date] you wrote: "I ask you to please tell me why I should give my money to your organization for emergency care, when my situation was neither handled with urgency nor care?" In response to that question I must state that although it is clear that you were less than satisfied with your encounter at our facility, the fact remains that you were triaged, checked in, examined, diagnosed and treated within a time frame consistent with that of emergency rooms within the community. You were prescribed medication, provided with names of local primary care providers, and given information on the diagnosed condition.

Based on my review I must decline your demand that we reverse the charges associated with your visit.

Sincerely,

[Name]
[Title]

Rewrite

[Date]

[Name]
[Address]

Dear ______________,

[Name], the director of emergency services forwarded your complaint and request for retraction of your bill to me for review. I appreciate you sharing your concerns with us. We take every complaint seriously and believe it is the best vehicle for fulfilling our mission for high quality of care for every patient.

I carefully reviewed your complaint, including investigating the time at which you arrived and were discharged as well as speaking with the physician involved. Following are the results of my investigation.

You presented to the emergency department on [date]. Our staff assessed your symptoms and noted you had stable vital signs. Our emergency department staff registered you. You stated that you were sent to the waiting room rather than an examining room. I understand that this concerned you.

I apologize that staff did not clearly explain our process. We will take this opportunity and ensure that future patients are carefully and clearly informed about our process and possible waits. While we do seek to provide care in an expeditious manner, we do so by severity of condition. If a patient came in after you and was determined to have a condition that was more serious, that patient would be seen before you.

Our records do indicate that Dr. [name] examined you and prescribed a course of treatment. You were discharged at two hours and 19 minutes from the time you were checked in. Although I can understand that this seemed a long wait, especially if our process was not clear to you, this is actually slightly less than the average amount of time to wait for non-critical treatment in an emergency room.

I am sorry that you felt that Dr. [name] was disrespectful and lacked compassion. Please feel free to contact me to elaborate about what specifically Dr. [name] said or did that was disrespectful. We sincerely wish to ensure that all patients are treated with courtesy and respect. This is a part of [name] Hospital's mission.

In your letter to Mrs. [name], dated [date] you requested a retraction of your bill because you were dissatisfied with our care. Again, I apologize that our care did not meet your expectations. However, we did perform the appropriate actions (triaged, checked in, examined, diagnosed and treated) within a time frame consistent with that of emergency rooms within the community. Therefore I am unable to retract your bill due to hospital policy.

[Consider another good will gesture such as a gift certificate if appropriate.]

We hope you are doing well and you are satisfied with the improvement measures we have taken. Should you have further concerns please contact me [name] at [telephone number].

Sincerely,

[Name]
[Title]

CHAPTER 14

What to Write—Sample Template Letters

CHAPTER 14

What to Write—Sample Template Letters

First response—verbal, in person, or written

This chapter contains sample template letters for many typical situations in which you will need to respond to patient concerns. Consider using these templates as a guide for writing your own specific letters. Please also use any letters within this book as a guide.

Letter style

[Header]
[Name]
[Address]

Dear ___________

I am writing in response to the [letter/call/comment] that [enter department or individual receiving the letter] received from you. In this letter you outline concerns about the care you received while you were a patient at [enter facility unit etc.] this past [insert date]. Your concerns were [enter specifics about the situation and the departments and/or services of concern].

I was very sorry to hear that your experience at [Organization name] was less than satisfactory. I have looked in to each of the issues that you identified and I have shared your comments with the [name and title of appropriate person]. [State next step if any or closure comment about concern.]

Thank you for bringing these issues to our attention. Although we cannot change the experience that you had with us, your observations and comments will help us in our continuing efforts to improve the care that we provide. We hope, that should the need arise, you will allow us the privilege of serving you again in the future.

Sincerely,

[Signature and title]

Memo style

Complaint:

[State complaint, including name of complainant, to whom the complaint was directed, date complaint was made and received, any names involved in receiving or handling the complaint, complainant's requested action or any third-party requested/required action, and any other relevant specifics.]

Summary of the issues that were reported:

[State the specific complaint, including as many relevant details as you can.]

[Keep a log of all contacts, verbal or written, and attempts to contact, the complainant and anyone involved in the complaint.]

Investigative findings per review of medical record and interviews with all departments involved:

[List all actions taken to investigate and resolve this complaint.]

[Close when the complaint is resolved and document the closure.]

Follow-up letter template

General apology

[Date]

[Name]
[Address]

Dear ________________,

Thank you for your letter of [date]. We take such concerns seriously at [name of hospital]. I appreciate being given the opportunity to address your concerns relative to the quality of care received by [patient] while at [name of hospital].

[Customize based on circumstances: I understand that since your meeting with __, you were contacted by ___, who is the ____]. I hope some of the issues were resolved during this conversation. We deeply regret and apologize for failing to meet your expectations of us as a health care provider. I am convinced that each of the individuals involved care about [patient's name] well-being and work hard to provide [him/her/you] with the best possible care.

All of us express our thoughts and feelings differently, but it is essential as health care professionals that we put the physical, emotional, and spiritual health of our patients and their families as our central focus at all times. Please accept our apology for any part we may have played in the [situation]. We are working daily to improve these elements of our service.

I hope that [patient's] recovery is progressing smoothly and that we can remain your hospital of choice for the future.

Sincerely,

[Name]
[Title]

Status of investigation

Acknowledgement of concern and explanation of next step

[Date]

[Name and Address]

Dear_______________,

Thank you for bringing to our attention your experience at [facility]. I know it can be difficult to discuss and sometimes even more difficult to report issues related to the medical care you received during your hospitalization. Nonetheless, such reports help us identify areas that need attention and improvement.

It is our goal to provide every patient with the best possible medical services. [Name of person and person's title] will be reviewing your concerns regarding the medical care that you received. I am truly sorry about your experience at our facility. If I can be of further assistance to you in this matter, I can be reached at [telephone number].

Sincerely,

[Name]
[Title]

Explanation of findings and next step or action

[Date]

[Name]
[Address]

Dear ________________,

Thank you for contacting us with your concerns [specify concerns and name facility, include a date of care and date concerns received]. Your complete satisfaction is very important to us. We appreciate your comments. Your input gives us the opportunity to review our services and make changes where necessary.

In addressing the particular concern, we have found that [describe findings] and plan to [describe next step or action to take].

We regret that you had this experience and we have followed up on your comments and have thoroughly discussed the situation with the appropriate personnel. It is our commitment to do everything possible to ensure that this situation does not occur in the future.

Thank you again for taking the time to share your concerns. If I can be of assistance in the future, please call me at [telephone number].

Sincerely,

[Name]
[Title]

Resolution letter

Result of investigation and corrective action (if any)

[Date]

[Name]
[Address]

Dear ___________,

I have been asked on behalf [name and title] to respond to your phone call describing the care that you received from us [date]. Thank you for taking the time and effort to let us know about your concerns and giving us an opportunity to address them with you. Our mission is to at all times, provide quality, compassionate care to our patients. Your description of a quite different experience is very concerning to us.

It is my understanding that your concerns include the following:
[List issues]

- Investigation of Issue #1 Findings [from chart, interviews, etc.]
- Investigation of Issue #2 Findings [From chart, Interviews, etc.]

[Include any corrective action taken or performance improvement measure implemented.]

Lastly, I personally apologize to you for your not receiving the level of care and service you expected. It is our aim to meet and exceed your expectations for quality health care. Thank you again, knowing that your input helps us to continually make improvements in the quality of our service.

Sincerely,

[Name]
[Title]

In a case of error or fault

[Date]

[Name]
[Address]

Dear _________________,

Thank you for sharing information about your experience at [name of hospital]. We sincerely regret our service did not [meet or exceed] your expectations. Your opinion is very important to us and in an effort to correct and improve our service as we discussed [Note in brief summary format the corrective actions that have been taken i.e.: staff has been counseled, an educational program is being held, the equipment has been taken out of service and sent for repair, engineering is addressing a corrective plan of action, etc.]

We are committed to continual improvement of our service and thank you again for taking the time to express your concerns. You have been helpful in assisting us to improve our performance.

We hope [you or reference your family members] are satisfied with the corrective measures we have taken. Should you have further concerns please contact me [include your telephone number and/or e-mail] or [include any other contact names and information].

We want to be [your or your families'] health care system of choice. In the future we want to continue to serve you and your family with the highest possible quality of care.

Sincerely,

[Name]
[Title]

Letter when complainant does not respond to telephone calls and/or letters

Unable to reach complainant by telephone

[Name]
[Address]

Dear ____________,

I received your concern regarding [summary of complaint] on [date]. I have attempted to call you during the day, but have unfortunately not been able to reach you. I have [state any action taken or current status of complaint. However, at this point we do need to follow-up with you in order to continue investigating your concern through our process. Would you please contact me at your earliest convenience to let me know the best way and time to reach you? You may contact me by telephone or by e-mail. [Insert specific contact information or attach a business card.]

I appreciate you taking the time to communicate your concern. At [name facility], we take a vested interest in your satisfaction with our services. I trust I will be hearing from you soon.

Sincerely,

[Name]
[Title]

SECTION VI

MANAGED CARE LETTERS

SECTION VI CONTENTS

CHAPTER 15

Replies: How Managed Care Responds to Patient Complaints

CHAPTER 15

Replies: How Managed Care Responds to Patient Complaints

Response to requests to change PCP

These are letters from insurers to patients. Most surround billing and financial issues. It's very important in these letters to avoid assumptions—don't use acronyms or abbreviations because the patient may not know what they mean; use extra details and provide feedback on "why" you've come to the conclusion you have. Another key: Blend facts with apology in cases when the patient or family member has gone through some sort of hardship.

Issue: In-network physician too far

[Date]

[Name of Recipient]
[Address]

RE: [Subject line and/or case number]

Dear ___________,

This is a follow up to the complaint you filed to [name of insurance company] through the sales department on [date].

The issue you brought to our attention was the fact that you needed to see an orthopedic doctor. The one you were referred to practices in [city name] [doctor's name], which poses as an inconvenience for you in that it is too far for you to travel. You found an orthopedist in [city name] [second doctor's name] who is contracted with [name of insurance company] and since you live in [city name] you feel that this doctor would be more appropriate for you.

While [name of insurance company] recognizes the fact that there are contracted specialists whose practices are more conveniently located to patients than the specialist their PCP (primary care physician) is referring them to, the in-network benefits on this policy are based on physician networks rather than location. When a patient is referred to a specialist, that specialist needs to be within the network of the patient's PCP. One of the reasons why PCPs refer their patients within their own network is to help the PCP coordinate and maintain the quality of a patient's care.

This leaves two options available. The first option is to change your PCP to a doctor who would refer you to [second doctor's name]. We have discussed PCPs who are affiliated with the same network as [second doctor's name].

The other option is to utilize your out-of network benefits. If a POS (Point of Service) plan member were to receive specialty care through a [name of insurance company] provider without a referral from his or her PCP, that service would be considered out-of-network. The POS plan allows one to utilize the services from out-of-network providers without a referral. If the patient chooses to receive care out of the physician network of his or her PCP then the monetary responsibility of the patient is the deductible and/or coinsurance.

Thank you for your inquiry and I hope I helped clear up the specifics of how to receive specialty care at an in-network level on your POS plan. If for any reason you need to contact me you can reach me directly at [telephone number]. If you prefer, my e-mail address is [e-mail address].

Sincerely,

[Name]
[Title]
[Name of insurance company]

Issue: PCP mix-up results in denied claim

[Date]
[Name of recipient]
[Address]

RE: [Subject line and/or case number]

Dear ___________,

I am writing as a follow up to the issue you brought to my attention in the Complaints Department at [name of insurance] on [date].

The issue was regarding our records showing the wrong primary care physician (PCP) for your son [name]. You indicated that you contacted the call center at [name of insurance] about a year ago to change his PCP from a [name of former PCP] to a [name of current PCP]. Recently, you began receiving a bill for services with [name of specialist]. You were told that there was no referral from [name of patient] PCP and therefore the claim would not be paid.

Through my investigation, I have discovered that [name of current PCP] referred [name of patient] to [name of specialist], however, [name of insurance] still had [name of former PCP] on file as [name] PCP. This is why the claim was denied. There are seven dates of service that have been denied payment because of this PCP discrepancy. Those dates with [name of specialist] are [range of dates].

There is also a bill from [name of current PCP] that has also been denied. The date of service for this bill is [date]. There is a denial for a date of service of [date], with a [name of specialist]. These claims have all denied for no referral.

The claims for dates of service [dates] with [name of specialist], that were referred by [name of current PCP] and paid by [name of insurance], should not have been paid since doctor other than the one that was [patient's name] PCP referred them.

As of [date], [patient's name] has been assigned to [name of current PCP] as his PCP. As a one-time exception, I have adjusted all the above-mentioned unpaid claims to pay. The claims for [date], and [date], will remain paid. Whenever you change your PCP, you can expect a new [name of insurance] identification card to arrive in the mail within 7-10 business days. If you do not receive one or if the information on the card is incorrect, please contact [name of insurance] to let us know.

Please do not hesitate to call me if you have any questions or wish to discuss this further. You can reach me at [telephone number] or [e-mail address].

Sincerely,

[Name]
[Title]
[Name of insurance company]

Mishandled claims

Issue: Delay in reimbursement

[Date]

[Name of recipient]
[Address]

Dear ____________,

Thank you for your recent phone inquiry. In light of the sheer volume of claims in question, I have decided that it would be prudent to produce an itemized list of your family's claims for you. You will find enclosed a sheet for each member of your family. All claims that you or a provider submitted to [name of insurance] are included. Each list includes all claims from your current [name of insurance] account [number] and your previous [name of insurance] account [number].

I understand your concern about receiving prompt reimbursement for medical services that you pay for out-of-pocket. I apologize for any mishandling of your claims that has occurred in the past. My hope is that these lists will help you reconcile what you have and have not received payment for. Please be assured that I am giving 100% to make sure that every one of your claims that comes to [name of insurance] is processed in a timely manner.

I would also like to point out that most of the claims that [name of insurance] has processed as direct reimbursements to you, have been paid and the checks have cleared. If after reviewing these lists you find that there are still unresolved issues, please contact me and I will be happy to help you resolve them.

Again, I apologize for delay in payment and for any inconvenience this matter has caused you. If I can be of any further assistance in this matter, please don't hesitate to call me toll-free at [phone number], Monday through Friday between 8:30 AM and 5:30 PM.

Sincerely,

[Name]
[Title]
[Department]

Issue: Appeal for claims reimbursement

[Date]

[Name of recipient]
[Address]

RE: [Subject line and/or case number]

Dear ______________,

I am following up on the letter that you sent to the appeals coordinator at [health insurance (HI)] dated [date]. Because I am the complaint coordinator for [HI], the letter was forwarded to me for review and response.

In your letter you indicated that you contacted [HI] on several occasions to resolve your claims for services received at [hospital name]. The letter indicated that you were told that these claims would be paid as in-network claims.

In [year], [hospital name] was a contracted mental health provider. [Name of doctors] were both contracted through the hospital but were not contracted as independent physicians. The bills appeared to be from independent practices, which is why they were paid with amounts toward deductible and coinsurance.

I did verify that the services did take place in the outpatient behavioral department at [Hospital name]; therefore I had the claims adjusted to pay at the in-network rate. The dates of service include [range of dates] from provider [name of doctor]. [Range of dates] with [name of second doctor] were also adjusted to pay at the in-network rate. I will monitor the claims in the system and notify you when a check number is assigned to them.

Thank you for your letter and I apologize for any inconvenience this matter has caused you. If you would like to contact me to discuss this further you can reach me at [telephone number].

Sincerely,

[Name]
[Title]
[Company]

Response to termination date error or oversight

Issue: Early termination from plan

[Date]

[Name of recipient]
[Address]

RE: [Subject line and/or case number]

Dear ____________,

This letter is in response to the letters you sent to the attention of the CEO and to the member appeals department at [name of insurance] both dated [date]. The letters were forwarded to me in the complaints department on [date].

In your letters you indicated that because of an error made by [subscriber agent's name], the subscriber of this plan, you were terminated from the plan a month before the termination date you intended. You also stated in your letter that you knew you had a biopsy scheduled in [month] and expected that you would still be enrolled with [name of insurance] until [later date after month] when your other insurance took effect.

Through my investigation I have discovered that the error was not made by [subscriber agent's name] but by the employer group itself. I was forwarded a copy of a request from [name of employee] to [name of second employee] at local [name of insurance] that specifically asks for a [date] termination date. The termination form we received by the Local [name of insurance] specifically indicates that the effective date of your termination is [date] meaning the last day of coverage is [earlier date].

[Name of insurance] has a contract with the Local [name of insurance] as an employer group. The employer group must initiate any changes made in the enrollment or termination of an employee. Therefore, [name of insurance] cannot change the enrollment or termination dates of an employee of that group based on anything except what we receive by the group itself. The Local [name of insurance] has a 90-day period to amend their request to enroll or terminate an employee retroactively.

I contacted the Local [name of insurance] and spoke with [name of second employee] who indicated that the [date] she displayed on the termination form was an error and that the date should have been [date]. I have brought this information to the attention of our account services department and they have approved coverage for you during the month of [month and year].

The claims for [month and year] will now be adjudicated and paid.

I am glad I could be of assistance in updating your policy and absolving your responsibility of this claim. If you would like to contact me to discuss this further you can reach me directly at [telephone number] or toll free at [toll free telephone number]. If you prefer, my e-mail address is [e-mail address].

Sincerely,

[Name]
[Title]
[Name of insurance company]

Issue: No physicians available prior to termination

[Date]

[Name of recipient]
[Address]

RE: [Subject line and/or case number]

Dear ____________,

Thank you for the letter you sent to the appeals department at [name of insurance company], your letter has been forwarded to me in the complaints department.

In your letter you indicate that you injured your knee within a day prior to moving from [state to state]. There were no available openings for you to receive an MRI needed to accurately identify your injury. You were told that you could have the test performed in [second state]. When you arrived in [second state] you went to the emergency room as directed, however they could not schedule you for the proper test until after the [holiday] weekend.

The test was performed on [date]. Your policy with [insurance company name] was terminated on [earlier date]. Although you had other active health insurance at the time, you indicated that they considered your injury to be a pre-existing condition and therefore would not pay for it.

As we discussed, [name of insurance company] does not pay for follow-up service outside the area without the proper referrals, nor are we obligated to pay any bills that are incurred after the termination date of a member. However, since the facility needed to properly diagnose your condition was unavailable at the time of the injury and because you were scheduled to move immediately after the injury it is obvious that you could not be subject to these types of constrictions. Therefore, the cost of the diagnostic test performed on [date] will be honored by [name of insurance company].

As we discussed, you will pay the full price of the procedure and I will set the system up to reimburse you for the cost of the service. The reimbursement process takes six to eight weeks.

I am glad I could help you resolve this issue. Thank you again for your letter. If you need to contact me for any reason, you can reach me at [telephone number].

Sincerely,

[Name]
[Title]
[Company]

Response to claims and benefit explanation

Issue: Prescription not filled and reimbursement

[Date]

[Name of recipient]
[Address]

RE: [Subject line and/or case number]

Dear ___________,

This letter is in response to the telephone call you made to the member services department at [name of insurance company] on [day and date]. As you may recall, the phone call was transferred to me in the complaints department.

During that call, there were two separate issues you wished to discuss. The first was regarding your prescription medication through [name of current pharmacy]. You indicated that you felt as though you were caught in the switchover from [name of former pharmacy] to [name of current pharmacy] and that your order was lost. This forced you to go to the pharmacy and purchase a 10-day supply of both [name of medications]. The combined price for these medications was [state amount].

The other issue you need a resolution on is regarding the reimbursement of eyeglasses you originally purchased through [name of insurance] in [name of town]. You indicated that you have been waiting quite some time for your reimbursement.

As a result of my investigation on the issue with [name of current pharmacy], I have discovered that on [date], your request for medication was received by [name of current pharmacy]. The request was filled and sent on the following day [date]. It never arrived to its destination due to an error on your address made by [name of current pharmacy]. The prescription medication was returned to [name of current pharmacy] on [date].

Fortunately, you contacted [name of current pharmacy] on [date] to inquire about the status of your medication. At that time, [name of current pharmacy] recognized their error and sent you your medications overnight delivery. Because of this error, I have arranged for [name of current pharmacy] pharmacy to give you a credit on your account in the amount of [state amount].

I have spoken to the manager in the [name] Optical shop who indicated that the reimbursement for your eyeglasses has been processed. You should receive your reimbursement within the next four weeks. The check number is [number] and it is for [state amount].

I apologize for any inconvenience this matter has caused you. If you would like to contact me to discuss this further you can reach me at [contact information].

Sincerely,

[Name]
[Title]
[Company]

Issue: Request for additional visits with specialist

[Date]

[Name of recipient]
[Address]

RE: [Subject line and/or case number]

Dear _____________,

I am writing to follow-up on the issue you brought to the attention of [name of insurance company] on [date] through the [name of insurance company] corporate Web site.

The issue was regarding your request to be certified for additional visits prior to receiving the full outpatient mental health benefits as stated in your Summary of Benefits (SOB). In your letter you also indicate that you were told by [name of insurance company] that you would need to appeal any denial over the benefit maximum.

The first thing I would like to establish is the current outpatient mental health benefit associated with your plan, then I will explain the process for receiving outpatient mental health benefits beyond your benefit limit.

The basic mental health benefit on the plan through [name of group employer] is for up to 24 individual therapy visits per calendar year (at a $15 co-payment each visit), and/or up to 25 group therapy visits per calendar year (at a $10 co-payment each visit). There is a 25 visit per calendar year maximum for combined individual and group outpatient therapy visits. To be covered by the plan these services must be obtained through [name and contact telephone number of mental health care subcontractor] who will assist you by finding a contracted provider and by arranging the services you require. [Name of mental health care subcontractor] is the third-party administrator for the [name of insurance company] behavioral health benefits. It is important to keep [name of mental health care subcontractor] informed of the care a [name of insurance company] member is receiving for tracking purposes.

Once an [name of insurance company] member has met the 24 visit individual outpatient therapy benefit maximum, that member's [name of insurance company] contracted mental health provider will need to contact [name of mental health care subcontractor] and speak to a care manager to initiate the review process for a benefit exception. If the member's diagnosis is a biologically based mental health illness and the [name of mental health care subcontractor] care manager deems additional outpatient mental health services to be medically necessary, a benefit exception will be approved for a set number of visits. When the additional authorized visit limit has been reached, the process will need to begin again. Once again, this process needs to begin after a plan member has met his or her annual benefit limit.

I would like to apologize for the misinformation given to you by a representative of [name of insurance company]. Waiting for a denial to file an appeal is not the [name of insurance company] preferred process for gaining authorization beyond the benefit limit of your plan.

If you would like to contact me to discuss this further you can reach me at [insert contact information].

Sincerely,

[Name]
[Title]
[Company]

Using the Files on Your *How to Resolve Patient Complaints to Manage Risk* CD/ROM

The following figures are included on your, *How to Resolve Patient Complaints to Manage Risk* CD/ROM:

Figures

Filename	*Description*
Fig2-1	Figure 2.1 Sample Privacy-Related Complaints Log Entry (editable file)
Fig2-2	Figure 2.2 Sample Privacy-Related Complaint Investigation Record (editable file)
Fig2-5	Figure 2.5 Sample Privacy Complaint/Concern Letter: Privacy Issues (editable file)
Fig2-6	Figure 2.6 Sample Privacy Complaint/Concern Letter: Notice of Privacy Practices (editable file)
Fig3-1	Figure 3.1 Heritage Valley Health System Administrative Policies and Procedures (PDF file)
Fig3-2	Figure 3.2 Sample Customer Comment Form from Heritage Valley Health System (PDF file)
Fig3-3	Figure 3.3 Sample Patient Complaint Process from Eastern State Hospital (PDF file)
Fig4-2	Figure 4.2 Sample Patient Complaint (PDF file)
Fig4-3	Figure 4.3 Sample of Intake Data Form (PDF file)

Letter Templates

1-letter	First response: Letter style (editable file)
1-memo	First response: Memo style (editable file)
followup	Follow-up letter (editable file)
apology	General apology (editable file)
acknowl	Status of investigation letter: Acknowledgement of concern (editable file)
explanat	Status of investigation letter: Explanation of findings (editable file)
result	Resolution letter: Result of investigation letter (editable file)
fault	Resolution letter: In case of error or fault (editable file)
unable	Unable to reach complainant letter (editable file)

To adapt the sample forms and policies and procedures to your own facility, simply follow the instructions below to open the CD. Each file is labeled with the figure number referenced in the book.

If you have trouble reading the forms, click on "View," and then "Normal." To adapt the forms, save them first to your own hard drive or disk (by clicking "File," then "Save as," and changing the system to your own). Then change the information enclosed in brackets to fit your facility, and add or delete any items that you wish to change.

Installation instructions

This product was designed for the Windows operating system and includes Word files that will run under Windows 95/98 or greater. The CD will work on all PCs and most Macintosh systems. To run the *How to Resolve Patient Complaints to Manage Risk* sample files CD/ROM, take the following steps:

1. Insert the *How to Resolve Patient Complaints to Manage Risk* CD into your CD/ROM drive.
2. Double-click on the "My Computer" icon, next double-click on the CD drive icon.
3. Double-click on the files you wish to open.
4. Adapt the files by moving the cursor over the areas you wish to change, highlighting them, and typing in the new information using Microsoft Word.
5. To save a file to your facility's system, click on "File" and then click on "Save As." Select the location where you wish to save the file and then click on "Save."
6. To print a document, click on "File" and then click on "Print."